LIZ EARLE'S

Dry Skin and Eczema

LIZ EARLE'S

Dry Skin and Eczema

BⵯXTREE

Advice to the Reader

Before following any advice contained in this book, it is recommended that you consult your doctor if you suffer from any health problems or special condition or are in any doubt as to its suitability

First published in Great Britain in 1995 as *Liz Earle's Quick Guide to Dry Skin and Eczema* by Boxtree Limited,
Broadwall House, 21 Broadwall, London SE1 9PL
This edition published in Great Britain in 1996 by Boxtree Limited

The right of Liz Earle to be identified as Author of this Work has been asserted by her in accordance with the Copyright, Designs and Patents Act 1988

10 9 8 7 6 5 4 3 2 1

ISBN: 0 7522 0548 X

Text design by Blackjacks
Cover design by Slatter~Anderson

Printed and Bound in Great Britain by Cox & Wyman Ltd., Reading, Berkshire

A CIP catalogue entry for this book is available from the British Library

Contents

ACKNOWLEDGEMENTS

I am grateful to Sarah Hamilton Fleming for helping to produce this book. Also to the many doctors and dermatologists who have assisted with its research, especially Professor Nicholas Lowe, Professor Ronald Marks, Dr David Atherton and Dr Michael J Cork. I am also indebted to Rachel Dalton, Julie Fisher, Sue Steward and the talented team at Boxtree, and to Rosemary Sandberg and Claire Bowles Publicity for their unfailing enthusiasm and support.

Introduction

Dry skin and eczema are increasingly common problems. The exact reasons for this are unknown, but are probably linked to many factors including environmental pollution, diet, stress and genetics. As a sufferer myself, I am only too well aware of the extreme discomfort and torment that these skin conditions can cause. And, as a mother of two small children with eczema, I am also aware of the difficulties of treating the disease in childhood.

In recent years, many advances have been made in the treatment and diagnosis of severe skin conditions. We have heard about special skin care, steroid creams, exclusion diets, food supplements and even Chinese herbs. While as yet there is no single cure for dry skin and eczema, there is much that we can do to help control it. No matter how bad our skin, there are positive steps we can take to improve its look and feel. I hope you will find this book an invaluable reference book and asset in the search for smoother, softer and more comfortable skin.

Liz Earle

——— 1 ———

Dry Skin and Eczema

Skin is a very variable material and the texture and condition of the skin on our faces is very different to that on our legs. Even small areas of skin, such as the face, can vary dramatically in texture and condition; for example, the skin covering the forehead is often oilier than the skin covering the cheeks. Human skin is generally impermeable, meaning that it prevents moisture loss and bars the entry of damaging particles. If the surface layer is very dry and flaky, this reduces the effectiveness of the skin as a barrier, allowing unwanted substances to enter the skin which may damage the developing cells, causing water loss and further flaking. The result can be very dry skin, ie skin that chaps, flakes, peels easily and which reveals wrinkles earlier than normal or oily skin.

One of the first warning signs of dry skin is an uncomfortable feeling that the skin is taut, especially after washing. Another symptom of dry skin is itching and blotching as a reaction to certain clothes or creams. Dry skin is the most commonly suffered skin complaint in the UK and, according to a survey carried out by skincare product manufacturers E45, one-fifth of women suffer from dry facial and body skin, so let's see what the causes of this common condition are.

CONTRIBUTORY FACTORS
* extreme weather conditions
* indoor heating at home and at work
* frequent washing with soap and detergents
* an inherited tendency to develop dry skin

* insufficient production of sebum (the skin's oil)
* ageing
* contact with irritating and drying chemicals – often in the form of detergents

Dry skin can also be one of the early symptoms of eczema where dry, red patches of skin develop on the front of the forearms, behind the knees or on the calves. These patches of skin can become excessively dry so that the skin cracks open, causing great discomfort. It is vitally important to lubricate these dry areas of skin regularly. We will take a closer look at eczema later on in this chapter. First though, let us examine the structure of our skin and how it functions.

Our Skin's Structure

Water is essential to our survival and it amounts to 60 percent of our body weight. In an average person weighing 60kg, around 6,000ml of water are stored in the dermis, 120ml in the epidermis and 20ml in the outermost layer. The water present in the skin ensures that the skin's natural moisturising mechanism continues to function and any deficiency manifests itself in a feeling of dryness. We are probably more prone to developing dry skin during the winter as our skin is exposed to extreme weather conditions such as freezing wind and rain, as well as dry heat from indoor heating systems. If the air humidity falls below 85 percent, water evaporates through the epidermis into the atmosphere, but if the air humidity is maintained above this level the stratum corneum (the uppermost layer) tends to draw moisture in from the atmosphere.

THE EPIDERMIS
These outer layers of skin are responsible for the production

and maintenance of the surface layer of our skin, acting as a protective barrier for the body. The epidermis prevents water loss and provides a little protection against ultraviolet (UV) damage from the sun and bacterial infection.

Cell renewal

To function properly, the outer layers of our skin are continually renewed. Every day the outer layer of skin dies and a new layer of cells is produced in its place by a process known as cell division. This outer layer, the stratum corneum, is particularly important in maintaining the skin's moisture (each square inch of human skin contains about twenty million cells).

Cell renewal, creating a strong protective barrier, is especially important for dry skin conditions such as eczema. The cells in the stratum corneum are protected by a hydrolipidic film, made from a mixture of water, proteins and mineral oils. Cells are supported by lipids (fats) which protect them and help to bind them together. These elements are essential for maintaining the stratum corneum.

THE DERMIS

The dermis exists purely to support the epidermis and it is divided into two parts: the papillary and the reticular. The papillary layer lies directly underneath the epidermis, and nerve elements and blood vessels run through both skin sections. Body hairs grow within the dermis up through the epidermis, and sebaceous glands are usually found next to the roots of these hairs. The reticular part of the dermis contains connective tissue, below which lie fat, muscle and the main blood supply. There are three varieties of connective tissue fibres: collagen, elastin and reticulin and these determine the strength and flexibility of our skin.

The skin is the outside shell which we present to the world, and the condition of our skin determines our appearance. It has the important job of protecting our body from the harsh elements of nature and pollution, as well as being an important organ of detoxification. Much of our bodily waste is excreted through the pores of our skin as sweat, and if the pores are blocked by dirt and dead skin debris, then this necessary function will be inhibited. Blocked pores will also block the production of sebum, which is the skin's natural moisturiser. It is the job of the sebaceous gland to secrete sebum through the hair follicles all over our bodies, to lubricate the hair and skin. These glands can become overactive and cause acne and minor skin blemishes, but in dry skin conditions, the opposite is the case. Perhaps the most important role of the skin is to regulate our body temperature. It is responsible for dissipating any excess heat in order to prevent an increase in temperature. In cold weather our bodies try to prevent any loss of heat by decreasing the skin's blood flow, which is why the skin can appear white or even blue in cold weather. Similarly, when it is hot, the skin blood flow is increased making our skin turn red. Regulation of body temperature is one of the many functions of the skin often impaired in people suffering from eczema.

Just as our eyes are said to be the window to the soul, our skin reflects our physical and mental health. The condition of our skin is not affected merely by external factors such as wind, pollution and heating systems, but also by the health of our body hidden beneath its protective clothing. Our skin reflects our diet and lifestyle – if you have a poor diet, drink alcohol or smoke cigarettes, then your skin is over-exposed to toxins and will not be getting enough of the vital vitamins and other nutrients essential for strong, healthy skin. Many skin conditions are also exacerbated by diet; for example, eczema may be triggered by dairy produce or nuts. We will examine the relationship between diet and skin disorders in Chapter 5.

Our skin also reflects our emotional state and almost everyone will show stress through the skin. Again, many skin conditions, including eczema, are exacerbated by stress and emotional upsets. The condition of our skin itself can cause a great deal of stress and one in ten people with problem skin admit that it affects their confidence. The majority of us can be embarrassed by having a large spot on our faces, but dry flaky skin or eczema is more obvious and can cause far greater discomfort and embarrassment.

Skin Conditions

DRY SKIN

Human skin is 10–20 percent water by weight. If the water content drops much below 10 percent, the surface of the skin becomes dry and the protective water barrier in the upper level of the skin is no longer effective. As well as being a condition in its own right, dry skin can also be a symptom of other more serious skin conditions such as dermatitis, eczema and psoriasis, which afflict many people.

It is interesting to note that dry skin is more common in people with fair skin than in those with darker skin. It is a rare sight to see olive-skinned southern Europeans with dry, flaky skin. Dry skin can also be inherited, as can most skin conditions including eczema and psoriasis.

BABY SKIN

Most babies have beautifully soft, clear skin, but a baby's skin is also very thin and vulnerable. It contains very few lipids (fats) and oil glands which provide natural protection against dry skin. Babies can develop a number of distressing skin conditions.

Chapped facial skin

Dry, chapped, irritated skin can be caused by a combination of milk, food, saliva, cold winds and dry air. It is important to keep the skin clean after each feed by washing it with warm water, after which an emollient (moisturising) cream should be applied. It is also a good idea to keep a dry cloth or bib under the chin to prevent chafing.

Milk spots

Another common skin condition in babies is white spots on the face, known as milk spots. These are caused by overstimulation of the sebaceous glands by maternal hormones. There is no treatment for this condition; however, it will clear up of its own accord after a few weeks.

Infantile seborrhoeic dermatitis

One of the most common forms of this condition is cradle cap and it is reassuring to know that this is not as distressing for the baby as it looks. Cradle cap is also caused by overactive sebaceous glands which have been stimulated by the mother's hormones. It is a condition of the scalp that starts with an oily rash and then develops into yellowy crusted flakes of skin. Regular treatment with a special shampoo containing salicylic acid, available from a doctor, should clear the condition in about four to six weeks.

Seborrhoeic dermatitis may also occur in the nappy area, where the skin becomes red and sometimes scaly. The yeast germ Candida, which is responsible for thrush, is often present and this can be identified by round, red, scaly patches on the lower half of the trunk. You will need an antifungal preparation from your pharmacist or GP to treat this condition.

Nappy rash

This very common skin problem is caused by irritation from constant contact with the ammonia present in urine, as well as irritation from faecal material. A red, dry scaly rash appears on the buttocks and thighs and in severe cases ulcers may develop. Your doctor may prescribe protective creams and ointments but the most important method of prevention and treatment of nappy rash is to maintain scrupulous hygiene in this area:

* change your baby's nappies regularly as soon as they become soiled
* clean the area thoroughly using a gentle soap for sensitive skin, making sure that you carefully rinse off all irritating soap residues
* dry carefully and apply a protective barrier cream or, if needed, an antifungal cream
* avoid the use of plastic pants whenever possible and, if in a warm room, try to leave the nappy off for as long as possible to allow air to help heal the skin
* disposable nappies are preferable, although they are expensive and potentially bad for the environment. If you do use towelling nappies, make sure they are rinsed thoroughly, as residual detergent and antiseptics can cause irritation

ICHTHYOSIS

This common condition is characterised by dry, rough skin which can leave us looking and feeling like a scaly reptile. The skin covering the joints such as the knees and elbows in general is affected, and children between the ages of one and four are most at risk, with boys slightly more prone to developing the condition than girls. Severe scaling can impair the development of hair and nails, and sufferers usually show another sign of atopy (an inherited tendency to develop certain diseases), such as eczema, asthma or hay fever. There is no permanent cure for this skin condition, although regular use of a good moisturising cream and bath oils can help rehydrate the skin. Doctors may occasionally recommend the use of peeling agents such as alpha-hydroxy acids, found in milk, fruit and proteins, to reduce the surface flaking.

DRY SKIN AND THE ELDERLY

It is a sad fact that our skin deteriorates with age due to a number of factors. Our sebaceous glands produce less sebum, the skin's natural emollient, so that we have less protection against water loss. Reduced sweat levels also contribute to the dehydration of our skin. Not only does our skin become drier in old age, it is also depleted of collagen, a protein which supports the structure of the skin, causing our skin to wrinkle. Our skin's stores of the protein elastin also become depleted, making the skin sag, and the overall rate of skin cell renewal slows down in old age leaving our skin more prone to dryness and cracking and slower to heal. Other contributory factors to dry skin in old age are poor circulation and nutrition, anaemia and inadequate heating and clothing.

To prevent dry skin, avoid using soap; instead use oil-based cleansers on the face and bath oils. A word of caution: bath oils may make the bath more slippery, so use a bath mat or install bath rails to make getting into and out of the bath easier. Severe dry skin often causes itching (senile pruritus) which can be very distressing and uncomfortable. Scratching will merely aggravate the problem and may cause further inflammation and spreading of the condition. Apply a soothing emollient cream to replace lost moisture and to protect the skin against further moisture loss. Try to wear cotton next to the skin as this has a cooling, soothing effect on the skin whereas wool and many manmade materials may add to the itching. If the itching is very severe a doctor may prescribe oral antihistamines.

DERMATITIS

The skin normally performs its function as a barrier very effectively. However, if toxic substances penetrate the epidermis, the skin may become damaged and inflamed. This may be caused by an allergy or a simple irritation from chemical products such as detergents. There are many different types of dermatitis, but they all follow a similar pattern. When the skin first reacts to the attack of toxic substances, the dermis swells and becomes tender, red and hot. The skin is moist and swollen and can feel both itchy and painful, but fortunately this does not last long. Small blisters can form on the surface of the skin which may burst and cause weeping. After the moisture and swelling has died down, the skin is red, itchy and scaly, and a little crust may form. The itching can cause scratching, particularly in young children, and once the skin is broken it can easily become infected. If your skin develops dermatitis after it has been in contact with a new substance or material, then simply avoiding contact with this substance should ensure that you will not develop the rash again.

Although doctors can establish a great deal about a skin condition from a careful inspection, it is often necessary to perform additional tests to be absolutely certain of what type of dermatitis a patient has – or even to distinguish between dermatitis and other common skin problems such as psoriasis. A simple blood test will establish whether a person has atopic dermatitis and a more specialised test will look for specific allergies to cat hair, pollens or certain foods, for example. In some cases a dermatologist may remove a piece of skin to determine the exact form of dermatitis. Skin biopsies are not as unpleasant and painful as they sound and they can help avoid future discomfort from dermatitis by establishing the cause of the condition early on.

Patch tests are another method of finding out which substances cause an allergic reaction. After learning about the history of your problem and examining the skin, a specialist will decide which materials are likely to cause a reaction and will apply a dilution of the suspected substance to a patch of unaffected skin, usually on your back. This will be held in place with adhesive tape for forty-eight hours, after which the underlying skin is examined to see if it has reacted to the substance. The dermatologist may also test other substances which are likely to cause a reaction, such as nickel, chromium and rubber. Patch testing may seem incredibly simple but it is not a good idea to test yourself with substances which you think may be causing a reaction as things can go wrong – it is important to have accurate and reliable patch tests carried out by an expert. From the results of the patch test, the doctor will give you a list of the irritant substances, so that you can avoid further contact with these in the future.

Dermatitis is also linked to female hormone levels according to a study, carried out by skin specialists at Edinburgh University, of 150 women with dermatitis. The specialists observed that as many as one-third of the women experienced a worsening of their condition just prior to starting their monthly period. This was particularly true of women who suffered from premenstrual tension. Half the women in the group also claimed that their dermatitis worsened when they were pregnant, while one-quarter of women said that their condition had actually improved during pregnancy. Dr Daniel Kemmet and Dr Michael Tidman, who conducted the study, concluded that the results strongly suggest that female sex hormones play an important part in the condition of dermatitis in women. Other recent trials support this study and have revealed that women who are sensitive to such substances as nickel (commonly found in jewellery) also vary in the severity of their problem depending on the time of the month.

URTICARIA

This condition is more commonly known as nettle rash or hives and it is an allergic reaction that looks like a skin rash. It appears on the skin as acute inflammatory marks which itch and it is generally caused by a reaction to food, additives, drugs, something inhaled or the venoms of stinging and biting insects. Urticaria is an immediate hypersensitivity and a reaction can be noticed very quickly after exposure to the allergen. Approximately 10 percent of the population suffer from hypersensitivity in the form of hay fever, food allergies and certain types of asthma and eczema. More women are affected than men and any age may be affected, although it is more common in middle age. Urticaria is best prevented by avoiding the substance that you are allergic to, be it pollen or dairy products. The rash itself can be soothed with unmedicated creams and lotions such as calamine lotion.

ECZEMA

This terrible skin condition afflicts many people, especially children, and it can cause a great deal of stress and misery as well as discomfort to the sufferer. It is estimated that 5 percent of the British population suffer from eczema in varying degrees. Eczema and dermatitis are closely linked to each other as conditions of irritated and inflamed skin. Eczema is associated with problems which occur internally, while dermatitis is associated with external problems such as sensitisation. The word 'eczema' comes from the Greek word for 'boiling' and this is a fitting description. Eczematous skin is red, hot and itchy due to an increase in blood flow through the skin. This happens when capillaries in the dermis open up and allow blood to flow through them, and the blood is warm because it comes from deep within the skin. When an area of the skin is scratched or rubbed repeatedly, the outer layer becomes thick and scaly to protect against damage from further scratching. There are many types of eczema, but the most common are atopic, seborrhoeic, varicose and discoid eczema.

Atopic eczema

Atopy simply means that there is an inherited predisposition to allergies with a tendency to develop asthma, eczema and hay fever; the majority of eczema sufferers will have a family history of one or more of these conditions. Eczema sufferers do not normally develop the condition until after the first few months of life, and between 5 and 15 percent of school children have atopic eczema. However, atopic eczema is not just a disease experienced by children; it can appear for the first time during the teenage years or in adulthood. It can develop on a few small patches of skin, perhaps around the ankles or wrists, or on the whole body, and the skin becomes dry and itchy. This produces an automatic desire to scratch the skin, causing the body to release histamine which makes the skin red and inflamed. Sadly, there is no cure for atopic eczema although there are a wide variety of successful treatments. The condition tends to flare up and then quieten down and these bad patches can last for anything from one week to a number of years.

Although the cause of atopic eczema is not fully understood, it is known that it involves immunological reactions in the skin which are controlled by lymphocytes (a type of white blood cell) which enter the skin through the blood. The skin on the face, wrist, bottom, arms, elbows and knees can become inflamed, red, scaly and itchy, and with children there is the added danger of frenzied scratching causing a secondary infection. If this occurs, pus forms and the area will weep, causing great discomfort for the child and anxiety for the family. Happily, 90 percent of children with infantile or atopic eczema will grow out of it before they reach adulthood, although this is not much consolation to those enduring the agony of it at the time.

Emotional factors such as stress, worry and unhappiness exacerbate eczema, which explains why many adolescents experience a temporary worsening of the condition. (Parents should be aware that certain dispensations can be arranged for eczema sufferers with Examination Boards through the head of the school prior to taking exams.)

Some people may experience only very mild eczema on their arms, while others may be covered from head to toe with dry, cracked, itchy skin. This condition is very upsetting and often undermines the confidence of the sufferer, because it looks so unattractive. It can also restrict the types of career (such as hair-dressing, car mechanics and gardening) you wish to go into, if your condition is particularly severe, as exposure to certain industrial irritants can make eczema worse.

No one knows exactly what triggers atopic eczema but Dr David Atherton, Consultant in Paediatric Dermatology at Great Ormond Street Hospital, London, describes eczema as an 'ill-adapted response (by the immune system) to substances encountered in everyday life that we would normally regard as completely harmless'. In humans with healthy immune systems, foreign particles (antigens) enter the body and these are attacked by antibodies. The antibodies and white blood cells are our defence against attack from antigens found in viruses, bacteria and parasites. People with atopic eczema produce too many immunoglobulin 'E' antibodies which is why they often react to harmless foreign proteins in food when the rest of us do not.

Seborrhoeic eczema

The adult form of seborrhoeic eczema is usually a mild and often stubborn form of eczema which is generally found on the body where the sebaceous glands are situated, such as the scalp, face, upper part of the chest and between the shoulder blades. Adult seborrhoeic eczema is associated with an increased amount of yeast on the skin close to the sebaceous glands. Fair-skinned men between the ages of twenty and thirty are most at risk and the fine scaling of the scalp often causes excessive dandruff. The affected areas should be kept as clean as possible and hair should be washed regularly with a special seborrhoeic shampoo or, if less severe, with an antidandruff shampoo containing pyrithione zinc. There are a variety of lotions and skin cleansers formulated for this type of eczema, and exposure to sunlight often improves the condition.

Varicose (stasis or gravitational) eczema

This form of eczema tends to affect the elderly and is one of the drawbacks of walking upright rather than on all fours. The pressure in the veins of the legs is higher when standing than when lying down, and this can cause fluid to leak out of the tiny vessels resulting in swollen ankles and a red-brown discolouration, which may develop into leg ulcers. Eczema can appear on this site. Varicose eczema makes the skin on the lower legs spotty, inflamed, itchy and flaky. It is wise to seek medical advice when treating this condition, but using emollient creams and bath oils will help to reduce any dryness of the skin and steroids may be applied to the affected area to calm the inflamed skin. Unfortunately, those with varicose eczema often become allergic to the creams and other medications used on their legs, so try using only one remedy at a time. The ingredients which are most likely to irritate varicose eczema are preservatives, perfumes and lanolin so these should be avoided if possible.

Support stockings may also be of benefit. To prevent the onset of varicose veins, avoid putting on too much weight, and always wear support tights during pregnancy or at work if your job involves a lot of standing. Support tights should be put on before you stand up in the morning, so keep a pair close at hand. Even young men and women can develop varicose veins if they spend too much time standing up at work in jobs such as waitressing and retail work. If you spend the majority of the day on your feet, make sure that you put them up when you get home. For the best effect, lie on the floor with your legs resting against a wall at a 90° angle from the floor.

Discoid (nummular or coin-shaped) eczema

The cause of this common pattern of eczema is as yet unknown. It mostly affects the lower arms and lower legs and it appears as red, scaly or weeping skin, which is covered with a yellow crust when infected. Young adults, especially those who have had eczema previously, are most at risk from this form of the disease and, as with adult seborrhoeic eczema, it can be stubborn and difficult to get rid of.

Psoriasis

Over one million people in the UK suffer from psoriasis and the cause is as yet unknown, although we do know that at least one-third of reported cases have a family history of the condition. The familiar pink or red patches generally appear on elbows, have a silvery scaling surface and well-defined edge. Psoriasis is attributed to an increase in the thickness of the epidermis. In normal, healthy skin, the cell renewal process takes about three weeks to complete, but with psoriatic skin the process is accelerated to approximately one week, causing a build-up of cells on the skin's surface that are visible in layers. The top layer of the epidermis doesn't form into a normal keratin layer and the scales of keratin are easily dislodged, revealing twisted blood vessels beneath. White blood cells penetrate the epidermis, causing swollen blemishes, similar to spots, on the skin's surface. These generally appear on the palms of the hands and the soles of the feet, and dilated blood vessels dramatically redden the appearance of the skin.

Psoriasis usually occurs in early adulthood and, like all skin conditions, stress and emotional upsets make it worse. Small patches of psoriasis often clear up relatively easily when exposed to the sun. A far more chronic form of the condition, erythrodermic psoriasis, is much more serious and can be life threatening. The entire surface of the skin becomes hot, dry and red and if this happens to you medical advice should be sought immediately.

Psoriasis can spread over the skin completely as is the case with the leading character in Dennis Potter's television series, *The Singing Detective*, who suffered from psoriasis to such an extent that he was hospitalised. Psoriasis can impair certain bodily functions; for example, psoriasis of the finger nails can cause disability in the fingers.

One of the newest and most successful treatments for psoriasis is calcipotriol, a form of vitamin D prescribed to patients under the brand name of Dononex. This is available as a scalp solution, and as both a cream and ointment from your GP. These cannot be used on the face, but can be used elsewhere twice daily until the condition clears. One of the main advantages of this new treatment for psoriasis is the fact that it is clean to use, odourless and stain-free on both skin and clothes. As with the other skin conditions which we have examined, the dry, cracked skin of psoriasis can be rehydrated with the daily use of a rich emollient. One of the other treatments for psoriasis is coal-tar ointment, made from distilled wood or coal, which has some success in softening the hardened keratin. Unfortunately, coal tar can stain the skin and clothes. Steroid creams are also sometimes prescribed to psoriasis sufferers but one of the best cures is a good dose of sunshine. For this reason, doctors may prescribe a series of sessions under an intense sunbed. A more specific treatment involving exposure to UVA rays and the drug psoralen, known as PUVA therapy, is discussed in more detail on page 55.

Mineral salts have also been shown to be useful, and Middle Eastern doctors recommend their patients take regular dips in the Dead Sea. Our 'internal sea' is lymph and plasma and these feed our cells with vital vitamins and minerals. It has been discovered that seawater has a mineral content which is almost identical to that of the water surrounding our cells: including magnesium, sodium, potassium, phosphorus, iodine, calcium, zinc, copper, manganese, molybdenum, cadmium, iron and cobalt. Some beauty salons and health spas offer water therapy treatments where those suffering from eczema and psoriasis can bathe in sea water which is heated to a temperature of 38°C (100°F). This enables the trace elements to penetrate into the skin, feeding it with nutrients which help to eliminate toxins and build healthy skin cells.

Skin and the Sun

Sun can be beneficial to certain skin conditions, particularly psoriasis, but in excess it is very damaging. Our skin is attacked by both the UVA and UVB rays. The more dangerous UVB rays burn the surface of the skin and bring out a tan on our skin in hot weather. Sunburn can be very painful and in severe cases it may be accompanied by nausea and dizziness. If your skin is sunburnt, take a cool bath or shower to remove the heat from the skin, and then apply generous amounts of an unperfumed emollient to rehydrate the skin and soothe the soreness. Reapply the cream every couple of hours to calm any itching and to prevent the skin peeling too dramatically. It is also important to drink plenty of water to prevent dehydration. Medical attention should be sought if the skin blisters.

We are exposed to UVA rays the whole year round, even in winter. UVA rays are longer-wave ultraviolet rays and they penetrate deep into the dermis causing permanent damage and ageing and even, in some cases, skin cancer. It is therefore important to wear sunscreens throughout the year, even in winter, if you want to maintain young-looking skin. Many everyday skincare moisturisers contain sunscreens but if your skin is sensitive it is best to use products which contain natural rather than chemical sunscreens which can irritate the skin. Sunscreens with a high sun protection factor (SPF) should be worn in hot weather to stop the skin burning and prevent premature ageing. Make sure the sunscreens you buy protect against both UVA and UVB rays as many sun creams only protect against UVB rays. There is no such thing as a healthy tan, but the risks can be kept to a minimum. Those with fair skins will find that they burn faster than darker-skinned people and will always need maximum protection, between SPF 15 and 25. Avoid sunbathing during the middle part of the day when the sun is at its hottest and if you have got your heart set on developing a tan, despite all the risks, then build it up slowly. It is important to remember that ultraviolet rays penetrate cloud, water and flimsy clothing. Babies should be kept out of the sun and any exposed areas should be protected with sunblock. By far the best way to prevent sun damage and maintain youthful skin is to avoid the sun as much as possible and if you do want to have a darker skin tone, then there are a number of self-tanning lotions which are easy to use and create a very smooth and natural colour. See Chapter 2 for more on skin in the sun.

PHOTOSENSITIVITY

Certain skin diseases are photosensitive, meaning that they are sensitive to the sun and this can cause problems. Polymorphic light eruption is the most common of all the photosensitive skin diseases and it manifests itself in a number of ways. In its mildest and most common form it looks like a fine red rash or itchy, prickly heat, but it can also erupt into eczema-like lesions. This condition can occur at any time of sun exposure between half an hour and three hours, and it usually occurs in the spring when the sun is low and people have not built up any tolerance to the sun. Some people will find that their skin never develops any tolerance to the sun, and they will be prone to developing sensitive skin conditions like 'prickly heat' whenever their skin is exposed to the sun. Polymorphic light eruption is activated by both UVA and UVB rays.

Another skin disease caused by sun sensitivity is solar urticaria (hives) of which there are six different types. A reaction usually takes place within minutes of exposure to the sun, with the skin turning red and itchy with raised wheals. The areas of the skin which are normally covered up, such as the buttocks, tend to be affected, but thankfully the skin usually calms down and returns to normal within a few hours.

If you are prone to developing photosensitive skin conditions such as these, then you should stay out of the sun altogether.

—— 2 ——
Effective Skin Care

According to the skincare manufacturers of E45, dry skin is the most commonly suffered skin complaint. Fortunately, good skincare advice can make all the difference to those with both dry skin and eczema. As you may have already found, some types of skin creams and soaps can aggravate your skin, while others may soothe and give real relief from itching and flaking. Skin sensitivity is an increasingly common problem. Research indicates that around 60 percent of all women in Europe say they have sensitive skins. The key to effective skin care is knowing which products and treatments will work best for you and your family.

No matter what colour, type or condition of our skin, underneath the surface it all looks pretty much the same. Our skin forms a highly sophisticated barrier, through which it can release heat and sweat, but that keeps dirt, bacteria and pollutants out. Because our skin is designed to keep substances from penetrating the body it is almost impossible for skincare products to affect more than the uppermost layer of skin.

Emollients

The best group of products for dry complexions and for those with eczema are the emollients. These are gently occlusive, meaning that they lie on the surface of the skin and prevent water loss. They also help 'fill in the cracks' to some extent in dry, dehydrated skin. Top dermatologists agree that emollients are a vitally important part of skincare. Dr Nicholas Lowe, Professor of Dermatology in London and Santa Monica, USA, describes emollient creams and lotions as 'an integral part of any treatment of skin disease where the skin scales, such as eczema and psoriasis'. Another leading expert is Professor Ronald Marks, Head of Dermatology at the University of Wales College of Medicine. He describes emollients as being of 'immense value' to both patients and cosmetic users.

So how do emollient creams and lotions work? Emollients perform two tasks: they help to hydrate the skin by replacing the moisture lost from the surface and help the skin to retain water by leaving a barrier of oils on the skin, which protect against further moisture loss. Emollients are made with several different types of ingredients. For example, silicone is an emollient that leaves a protective film over the surface of the skin. Another example is petroleum jelly. This is frequently used as an emollient as it is good at adhering to the skin and is easy to spread. Most emollient creams or lotions are made from a mixture of water, waxes, fats and oils. They may include urea and glycerine, which have the capacity to increase the water content of the upper levels of the skin. Here, the skin absorbs water and swells with moisture supplied by an emollient cream. This swelling results in a smoothing of the skin's surface and is easily proved by viewing the skin under an electron microscope or by measuring the skin's surface profile in laboratory experiments.

EMOLLIENT INGREDIENTS
Glycerin
This is produced as a by-product of soap manufacturing and as a skincare ingredient it is a very strong water binder. In fact, it is so strong that it should not be used by itself by those with dry or sensitive skins. Glycerin can actually make dry skin worse over time as it not only attracts water from the atmosphere on to the skin, but it can also pull moisture away from the lower

levels of the epidermis, causing skin dehydration. However, glycerin is both useful and effective when combined with other ingredients in an emollient cream.

Hyaluronic acid

This ingredient is a water binder found naturally throughout the body. Hyaluronic acid can hold up to 400 times its own weight in water. Its molecules are quite large and so cannot penetrate the skin, but it is frequently used as an active hydrating ingredient. It is an expensive ingredient for manufacturers to use.

Lanolin

This is a good emollient and was first used by the Ancient Greeks as a skin soother. The renowned British herbalist Culpeper recorded how lanolin was obtained, but this process was not carried out commercially until the beginning of this century.

Lanolin is a unique blend of natural oils and waxes that form a protective coating on sheep's wool and skin. When sheep are shorn, the waxes are removed from the fleece and purified to produce lanolin. The good news is that lanolin is a natural and cruelty-free product. It is found in a surprising number of products, including baby oils, cleansers, moisturisers, barrier creams, lipsticks and shampoos. Some lanolin-based products are medically recommended and available on prescription to help relieve skin conditions such as psoriasis and eczema.

Despite the bad press it has received in the past, the number of incidences of allergy to lanolin is very low. Although some products are labelled 'lanolin free' there is no reason for the vast majority with dry skin or eczema to avoid it. The myth of lanolin allergy is due to the misinterpretation of the results of an American skin study over forty years ago, when lanolin wrongly gained a reputation for being the bane of sensitive skin. In fact, cases of lanolin allergy are extremely rare, and virtually unknown amongst the thousands of workers involved in its processing and refining. The renowned American dermatologist, Professor Albert Kligman, maintains 'lanolin is a marvellous material. We should begin to emphasise the benefits.'

Recent papers published in the *Journal of the Society of Cosmetic Chemists* have found that lanolin can penetrate the uppermost layers of the skin to provide intensive moisturisation. Studies show it may also help the skin to retain moisture deep within its cells. Purification processes for lanolin have also greatly improved over the years and purified forms are used in well-formulated skincare products. Emollients for dry skin and eczema tend to contain hypoallergenic lanolin, made by reducing the natural free fatty alcohols to below the allergenic threshold of 3 percent and by removing detergent and pesticide residues.

Mineral oil

This is a petroleum derivative and is refined to make it hypoallergenic. This means that it very rarely causes any allergy or irritation problems. On its own, mineral oil is very greasy (it is the same as baby oil) and does not sink into the skin. However, when formulated into an emollient it can be a useful ingredient to soothe irritated, dry and scaly skin. The other advantage is that mineral oil is very inexpensive and products that contain it tend to be economical to buy. This is especially important for those with clinical skin conditions who need to use large quantities of emollients on a daily basis.

Petroleum jelly

This has the same advantages and disadvantages as mineral oil. It is hypoallergenic and helps soothe very dry skin conditions. However, pure petroleum jelly (such as Vaseline) is highly occlusive, meaning that it contains heavy, large molecules that sit on top of the skin and form a sticky barrier. While this is good for preventing moisture loss, it does leave a greasy look to the skin and it is difficult to apply make-up with success. Although petroleum jelly does not cause blackheads in itself, it does prevent the hair follicles from releasing sebum and this can cause pimples beneath the skin. Water and sweat can also become trapped on the skin, causing a build-up of bacteria.

Petroleum jelly can be useful when used on its own to form a waterproof barrier or to shield the skin from contact allergens, such as nickel jewellery or fastenings. It is also used by doctors and dentists who are sensitive to latex gloves. By applying a small amount of petroleum jelly before wearing the gloves, a barrier is created between the skin and the latex, reducing contact and therefore the irritation.

Propylene glycol

This is the second most common ingredient in skin care after water. It penetrates the skin fairly rapidly and is used in a wide range of creams and lotions, including many make-up foundations. It absorbs moisture, acting as a solvent and wetting agent in liquid skin preparations. Propylene glycol is well tolerated by the skin although it may cause skin sensitivity in some.

Silicones

These are a group of raw materials derived from the natural mineral silica. Silicones may be used in skincare ingredients in the form of fluid oils, rubbers or resins. All are water-repellent and have good staying power on the skin. Silicones are used in a wide range of protective creams, hand and body lotions. They are also used in sunscreens, especially those designed to be waterproof or water-resistant.

Urea

This is one of the skin's own natural moisturising factors (NMFs) which help to preserve the water level within the skin layers, keeping it soft and supple. It has a high water solubility and attracts moisture. As we age, we tend to lose the ability to create these NMFs, which is one reason why older skin tends to be drier and taut. Fortunately, cosmetic chemists have been able to duplicate many of the natural moisturising factors in the laboratory including urea, which can be made from ammonia and liquid carbon dioxide. In fact, urea entered the history books as the first organic compound to be made artificially in a laboratory in 1828. This NMF is an excellent water binder and is also a keratolytic, meaning it can help to dislodge dead, loose skin cells from the surface of the skin. Urea is found in pastes and ointments prescribed for dehydrated skins. It is also used as a mild antiseptic and deodoriser.

EMOLLIENT BENEFITS

Using emollient creams and lotions on a regular basis not only smooths the surface of the skin, making it more attractive and comfortable, but also helps soothe the dry skin associated with inflammatory skin conditions. Minor fissures and cracks tend to close, sealing potential gaps for germs to enter, making the skin less tender and sore. Emollients also help to relieve the itchy nature of many dry skin conditions. Some research suggests that the ingredients in emollients reduce the inflammatory prostaglandins, hormone-like substances within the body responsible for causing skin irritations. Work by Professor Marks shows that some emollients help slow down cell division in the epidermis and that this probably contributes to the reduction in skin thickening and scaling that regular emollient users experience. Professor Marks comments that the paraffin hydrocarbon ingredients seem to be the most potent for producing this beneficial effect.

There are several reasons why emollients reduce itchiness. This is partly to do with their mild anti-inflammatory activity but, unlike corticosteroids, this anti-itch effect is also noticeable when the skin is not inflamed. This is due to the cooling effect caused by the evaporation of the water content.

Choosing Skin Care

Do not be afraid to use several different skincare products on a daily basis. Although it is true that some cosmetic creams can cause an irritation, the regular use of a cream and cleansing lotion or wash-off product which has been specifically formulated for dry and sensitive skin types is ideal. Using emollient creams and body washes on a daily basis not only keeps the skin soft and supple, but also disguises the appearance of skin flaking. It can also reduce the severity of skin chapping, cracking and bleeding. Studies by Dr Christopher Vickers, Professor of Dermatology at the Royal Liverpool Hospital, show that regular, daily use of a liquid emollient added to the bath water reduces the need to use steroid creams to control eczema. Patients noticed a 50 percent reduction in the quantity of corticosteroid cream used per week during the ten-month trial.

CLEANSING

To help preserve the protective film that covers the uppermost layer of skin which locks in moisture, avoid using soap and water as this will only strip the skin further. Most soaps are highly alkaline and can also upset the skin's naturally acidic protective film, causing irritation and flaking. Surprisingly, studies by the makers of Wash E45 show that 50 percent of eczema and 70 percent of psoriasis sufferers still cleanse their faces with skin-drying soaps. Soap does not cleanse the pores properly as it cannot dissolve the skin's own oil (sebum) or remove oil-based dirt and make-up. In addition, constant wetting and drying of the skin can worsen dryness. Keep the skin clean and clear by using an oil-based cleanser morning and evening. These can be used by all the family, and are also effective make-up removers. Apply a little to the skin, massage gently in, leave for a few seconds to allow the oil to dissolve the dirt, then wipe off with cotton wool or a damp flannel. Tissues are best avoided as they can scratch delicate skins. Gently pat dry with a towel.

Cleansing lotions and washes can be used in the bath or shower for all-over cleaning. Some emollients can be added to the bath and this is a useful way to soak the entire body. Washing in water alone dries out the skin, so medicinal bath oils have been developed to make bathing actively good for dry skin. Bath water should be lukewarm, not hot, as the sudden change of temperature will cause skin itching. After soaking in the water for about fifteen minutes (by which time the skin has absorbed some of the water), the moisture can then be sealed in with an emollient cream or body lotion.

As the substances present in hard water can dehydrate and irritate the skin it may be worth installing a water softener. This is fitted to the cold water supply in the house and softens the water to such an extent that a smaller quantity of skin-irritating detergents is needed for washing and laundry.

TONING

Having cleansed the skin, it may be useful to use a skin tonic or toner. Although not an essential part of our skincare routine, they can be useful to wipe away any remaining cleanser on the face. This is especially important in areas of hard tap water, where small mineral deposits may be left in the form of residue on the skin. When choosing a skin tonic, those with dry skin should avoid tonics containing alcohol. Some skin tonics contain soothing herbal extracts, such as aloe vera and comfrey (also known as allantoin), although people with eczema may find even those gentle toners too irritating.

MOISTURISING

Once the skin is clean, it can then be moisturised with a gentle emollient cream or lotion. Very dry skins may need several applications of emollient throughout the day, so it is useful to carry a small tube around with you. Even if your eczema or dry skin is under control, it is important to use a generous application of emollient cream every day. This is especially important when the weather turns cold as chapped skin tends to be worse in low temperatures and low relative humidity.

Studies involving British Army families found that 18 percent of the European patients were children with atopic eczema, whereas in Singapore fewer than 1 percent had the disorder. In Singapore the relative humidity is 90 percent – a convincing case for investing in a humidifier for the home. Additionally, a water spray or small canister of mineral water spray is useful for topping up your skin's moisture level throughout the day – especially if you live or work in a dry centrally heated or air-conditioned environment.

SKINCARE CHECKLIST

Bath oils – *Choose formulations from the chemist or pharmacy designed to cleanse without irritation. Add to the bath water to soften and clean the skin from top to toe.*

Wash creams – *The non-drying alternative to soap. Choose non-foaming, dermatologically tested preparations especially formulated for dry, sensitive skins.*

Emollient creams – *Use daily on the face, hands and body. Choose unperfumed, hypoallergenic creams to moisturise the skin deeply.*

Emollient lotions – *A lighter textured version of an emollient cream. Ideal for using on the body or for younger skin, including that of babies and children.*

Mild hydrocortisone creams – *A 1 percent hydrocortisone cream or ointment is available from chemists without prescription. This calms the soreness and itching of irritated skin for those with mild to moderate eczema. Also useful for treating contact dermatitis and reactions to insect bites. However, face creams should not be used for general skincare.*

Sunscreens – *Choose unperfumed products with a high sun protection factor (SPF) which protect against both UVA and UVB rays. Look for those made with non-chemical sunscreens to reduce the risk of skin irritation.*

It is worth noting that many emollient preparations, including creams and washes, are available on prescription. Ask your GP to advise you as those with eczema and clinically dry skin conditions can make a considerable saving.

Skin Care in the Sun

Most of us are well aware that the sun damages the skin. In terms of premature ageing and wrinkling, the sun is the skin's number one enemy. For this reason many creams and daily moisturising products contain a built-in sunscreen. Unfortunately, those with dry, sensitive or eczema-type skin conditions frequently find that these cause an allergic reaction or irritation. This is because many are allergic to chemical sunscreen ingredients. Para-amino benzoic acid, better known simply as PABA, has caused many allergic reactions. Although it is effective at filtering out the sun's UVB rays, many brands are now labelled as being PABA-free. However, those who are sensitive to PABA should also be aware of other chemical sunscreen ingredients, including padimate-O, padimate-A, cinnamates, homosalate, octyl salicylate and amyldimethyl PABA. These chemicals are all known to increase the risk of skin irritation, especially in those with eczema.

The physical type of sunscreen is best for dry and sensitive skins as they are far less likely to provoke an allergy or irritation. These sun blocks are based on inert powdered minerals, such as titanium dioxide, zinc oxide and ferric oxide. They work by forming a physical barrier against the sun that reflects or scatters the sun's rays and they block both UVA and UVB rays, although according to photobiology research they are slightly less effective at blocking the UVA rays than their chemical counterparts. Another drawback is that the powdered minerals can leave a slight chalky white residue on the skin, although scientists can now break down the minerals into microns, making them less visible and more versatile.

Plant oils such as sesame seed oil offer a limited form of natural protection and are often included in sunscreens to help soften the skin.

Antioxidant vitamins, such as vitamin E, are also included to prevent free-radical cell damage which can lead to cancer. Studies published in the *Archives of Dermatological Research* show that applying vitamin E to the surface of the skin helps prevent the skin from burning and may offer some help in soothing dry, itchy skin.

Sun blocks should be used over the top of an emollient moisturising cream.

SKIN CARE IN THE SUN CHECKLIST

* Choose a higher factor sunscreen than you think you will need. You can never have too much protection!
* Apply liberally for maximum benefit; rub in well so that the product is absorbed into the skin.
* Apply thirty minutes before stepping out into the sun.
* Choose a brand that does not contain chemical sunscreens. Look for products containing micronised titanium dioxide.
* Watersports enthusiasts and swimmers should choose a waterproof formulation.
* If you are playing sport in the sun always use a water-proof or water-resistant formulation.
* Avoid gel-based sunscreens as these have an alcohol base which may irritate sensitive skins when applied.

* Remember that water, sand and snow intensify the effects of the sun, reflecting the UV rays back at the skin.
* Re-apply sunscreen every hour throughout the day.
* Children and babies should wear total sunblock and be kept out of the sun as much as possible.
* Stay out of the sun between 11am and 3pm.

Fragrance Free

Perfumes and skincare fragrances are the largest single source of cosmetic allergies. Fragrances are used in virtually all skincare products, including moisturisers, cleansers and skin tonics. For those with dry and sensitive skins it is important to choose fragrance-free formulations. Even plant extract fragrances, including essential oils, may produce frequent allergies, especially in those who are very prone to allergic reactions.

The second most common category of cosmetic allergens is preservatives. These are necessary in all creams and lotions to prevent them from turning rancid on the shelf before we buy them. However, the anti-oxidant vitamins C and E can be used as natural preservatives instead. Preservatives also prevent harmful micro-organisms from contaminating the product. The most frequently used preservative complex in the cosmetics industry is parabens. Methylparaben and propylparaben are used in countless creams and cosmetics and are considered the safest forms to use. Used in small quantities these chemicals do not cause a problem for most of us. However, according to American dermatologist Dr Mark Lees, around 1 percent of the population may have a reaction to these preservatives.

Treatment and Prevention of Dermatitis

If you have sensitive skin and tend to develop rashes, then it is best to test cosmetics, moisturisers and cleansers on a small area of your skin before applying or using the product more liberally. Some cosmetic products will recommend this, such as hair dye instructions which often advise you to test the product on your skin to make sure that you are not allergic to any of the ingredients. It is best to apply the substance to a small area of unexposed skin, such as the inner elbow. Apart from avoiding strong, chemical products, the best method of preventing a reaction to irritants is wearing protective rubber gloves. If your hands react to the rubber, then use lined PVC alternatives or wear cotton gloves inside the rubber gloves and make sure that all gloves are washed regularly with a gentle detergent.

All dermatitis sufferers should take care when washing, avoiding the use of soap, solvents or abrasive cleaners. After drying the skin carefully, a good emollient moisturiser should be applied to prevent the skin drying out, minimising further cracking of the keratin layer. Look for skincare products which are designed to moisturise sensitive skins. For dry and itchy dermatitis, a hydrocortisone cream should be applied once or twice daily until the itching and dryness subsides, **but not for more than seven days as over-use can permanently weaken the skin**.

3

Conventional Treatments

Having examined some of the most common dry skin conditions and the best forms of skin care, it is time to look at the traditional methods doctors use when treating eczema sufferers and patients with other dry skin conditions. Children and pregnant women will need to seek special advice before taking any form of treatment. First, there are some basic measures which we can all take to look after our skin, and remember – care is the best treatment for dry skins! As we have seen, it is vitally important to moisturise the skin with emollients and bath oils on a regular basis to prevent the skin drying out completely and cracking. Everyone with dry skin conditions such as eczema should apply emollients regularly, at the same time as taking any other form of treatment that a doctor may prescribe.

Sadly, there is no permanent cure for eczema but there are plenty of positive measures that we can take to make it easier to live with. There are a variety of treatments which can improve dry skin, prevent and tackle skin infections and reduce inflammation and itching. Everyone's experience of eczema is different and it may take some time to find the best combination of treatments for you.

Those with dermatitis or eczema may develop an itchy, scaly scalp. Special coal-tar shampoos are available which help to soothe the itching and improve the condition of the scalp. These tar-based shampoos need to be used several times a week initially. They should be gently rubbed into the scalp, left there for a few minutes and then rinsed with warm, not hot, water. Tar pastes and creams can also be bought but these can be very messy to use and often stain the skin and clothes. Tar has been used to treat skin conditions for over a hundred years and it has a soothing, antiseptic and healing effect on the skin. You can also obtain coal-tar bandages on prescription which are useful for treating eczema on the arms and legs. Professor Lowe recommends these for many of the children with eczema he treats, although he concedes that the paste smells awful and tends to stain clothing and bedding.

Steroids

Corticosteroids are a group of naturally occurring hormones produced by the adrenal cortex (the outer portion of the adrenal glands which are situated near the kidneys). Corticosteroids are used widely in medicine either as replacement therapy in diseases which affect the natural production of steroids, or to suppress inflammation, allergy and other immune system responses. This latter use applies to the treatment of eczema and other inflammatory skin conditions. Each year corticosteroids are prescribed to around eight million people to treat common atopic conditions such as eczema, asthma and hay fever. They reduce the activity of white blood cells in the immune system which are responsible for causing inflammation, and thereby relieve the swelling and pain characteristic of many skin disorders.

The use of topical steroid creams and ointments for skin diseases has revolutionised the treatment of dermatitis, eczema, psoriasis and allergic rashes. Unfortunately, high dose topical steroids can have side-effects such as thinning of the skin, which may lead to the development of unsightly stretch marks. These first appear as red raised lines on the skin, which later fade into pale silver streaks, but they never vanish completely. This is caused by the steroids breaking down collagen and inhibiting fibroblasts from forming new collagen.

Topical steroids also suppress the body's reaction to local infection so that it is unable to fight infections properly. They should, therefore, be avoided if you have any skin infections such as cold sores, acne or athlete's foot. Highly potent topical steroids can have more serious side-effects if used for long periods of time, as a proportion of the steroids pass through the skin and enter the blood stream which can result in the same side-effects that occur when steroids are taken by mouth (see page 49).

Side-effects include a greater risk of developing diabetes and cataracts. Topical steroids should not be used for infected eczema or for mild forms of eczema although 1 percent hydrocortisone creams can be used to treat mild to moderate eczema.

AN A–Z OF TOPICAL STEROID OINTMENTS

Some topical steroids are far more potent than others. The more powerful formulations are used to treat very severe cases of eczema, while the mildest hydrocortisone creams are generally used to treat contact dermatitis and are also the main form of treatment for babies with atopic eczema.

Mildly potent

These topical steroids contain either 0.5, 1 or 2.5 percent hydrocortisone and they are generally safe for all age groups, although young children should only use them for short periods of time. Children under ten years of age should only use these creams under a doctor's direction. One percent hydrocortisone creams and ointments are available from chemists without prescription to treat contact dermatitis, mild to moderate eczema and insect bites. Even these very mild topical steroids should not be used on broken or infected skin. Eczema patients are sometimes prescribed hydrocortisone to keep their eczema under control.

HC45
Efcortelan
Hydrocortistab

Moderately potent

These can be obtained with a doctor's prescription. They contain slightly more potent forms of steroids and can be used to treat more severe dermatitis. They are also used to treat severe eczema in children and should not be used more than two to three times daily. Moderately potent topical steroids can be used on the face for short periods only.

> *Betnovate-RD – 0.025 percent Betamethasone valerate*
> *Eumovate – 0.05 percent Clobetasone butyrate*
> *Haelan – 0.0125 percent Flurandrenolone*
> *Synalar 1 in 4 dilution – 0.0025 percent Fluocinolone*
> *acetonide*
> *Stiedex-LP – 0.05 percent Desoxymethasone*

Potent

These can only be obtained with a doctor's prescription. They are generally considered to be unsuitable for children, although older children may be prescribed them to treat small areas of affected skin for short periods of time. They should not be used on the face without medical advice and should only be used elsewhere sparingly. If you are using highly potent topical steroids you should contact your doctor immediately if your skin condition deteriorates. Make absolutely sure that you do not exceed the recommended dose.

> *Betnovate – 0.1 percent Betamethasone valerate*
> *Diprosone – 0.05 percent Betamethasone dipropionate*
> *Locoid – 0.1 percent Hydrocortisone 17-butyrate*
> *Metosyn – 0.05 percent Fluocinonide*
> *Nerisone – 0.1 percent Diflucortolone valerate*

Preferid – 0.025 percent Budesonide
Propaderm – 0.025 percent Beclomethasone dipropionate
Stiedex – 0.25 percent Desoxymethasone
Synalar – 0.025 percent Fluocinolone acetonide

Highly potent

These should never be used to treat children or be used on the face. Again, it is very important that these topical steroids are not over-used as they can cause side-effects.

Dermovate – 0.05 percent Clobetasol propionate
Halciderm Topical – 0.1 percent Halcinonide
Nerisone Forte – 0.3 percent Diflucortolone valerate
Synalar Forte – 0.2 percent Fluocinolone acetonide

Dosage

To avoid applying too much topical steroid cream or ointment, a guideline, known as the Fingertip Dosing Unit, has been suggested to help eczema patients know how much they should apply. One strip of the ointment or cream, squeezed from an ordinary tube on to the tip of an adult finger down to the first joint on the finger, represents one unit. The National Eczema Society have a simple saying to help us remember that topical steroids should be applied thinly, while emollients should be applied thickly: 'spread steroids like Marmite, use emollients like marmalade!'

The number of units you need to apply to your skin depends upon the size of the area you are treating. The following doses of topical steroids are for adults with eczema, a very young child will need one-quarter of the adult dose and a four-year-old will need one-third of the dose:

* for one hand apply one fingertip unit
* for one foot apply two fingertip units

* for one arm apply three fingertip units
* for one leg apply six fingertip units
* for the front and back of your trunk (upper part of body) apply fourteen fingertip units

On the whole, the safety of using topical steroids has been demonstrated by decades of use and some of the side-effects can be avoided if they are used correctly. Creams containing 1 percent hydrocortisone are newly available from chemists without a prescription to treat mild to moderate eczema, contact dermatitis, including skin reactions to insect bites and stings. These creams work by controlling the fluid in cells, preventing them from building up and causing swelling, and also by tightening the blood vessels, restricting blood flow and so reducing redness. They also relieve irritation and soreness by suppressing inflammation, reducing associated itchiness and assisting in the natural healing processes of the skin. These are useful as they break the terrible itch–scratch– itch cycle, and help to reduce the habit of scratching, or unconscious scratching during the night.

Hydrocortisone preparations must not be used on the face or genitals unless under medical supervision. The anti-inflammatory action of these preparations is not immediately obvious and one or two applications should be made daily to the affected area for up to seven days. If the rash does not clear after seven days, then medical advice should be sought.

As with most treatments, frequent use of steroid creams can reduce their effect on the skin. To amplify the effect of these creams, a polythene film is sometimes used. First the topical steroid is applied, then a tubular bandage is placed over it with a plastic or polythene film put on top, which is firmly held in place by sticky tape. This technique is known as 'occlusion' and it works by increasing the hydration of the skin and enhancing the absorption of steroids through the barrier of the stratum corneum into the blood stream. Unfortunately, the improved absorption of the steroid increases the likelihood that it will damage the skin. Occlusion is rarely used to treat children as their ezcema is usually too widespread. However, it is often successful in treating small, persistent patches of eczema.

In some severe cases of eczema and other skin disorders, a dermatologist may advise that the patient be administered steroids orally. This can have much more serious side-effects than the topical use of steroids, if used regularly. When we take steroids orally, the adrenal cortex reacts by closing down its own cortisol production, which could be potentially dangerous as it is then unable to increase its production of cortisol in response to the threat of serious illnesses and infections. Our bodies become stressed when we are attacked by viruses and infections and we need to produce higher amounts of cortisol to enable our bodies to fight the infection.

However, the immunological suppressive effect of steroids is usually confined to those who are taking higher doses than generally used for eczema or asthma. Nevertheless, it is very important that patients are made aware of the serious side-effects of taking large doses of steroids for any length of time before they are prescribed them. There was a tragic case as recently as 1994 of a nine-year-old girl who died six weeks after being prescribed 80mg of steroids daily for a minor eye inflammation. She died of chickenpox because the steroids suppressed her immune system and made it impossible for her to fight the disease. Children on steroids usually cope well with infections except in the case of chickenpox, so if your child is taking steroids and is exposed to the disease, having never had it, you should consult your GP immediately. Adults taking steroids should also avoid coming into contact with people suffering from chickenpox and shingles.

Another worry is that taking steroids orally may reduce our resistance to the weakened viruses we are given when immunised against polio, influenza, hepatitis A and yellow fever.

Immunisations contain a tiny dose of the virus so that our immune system can build up a resistance to it. Those taking medium and high doses of steroids may be advised by their doctor not to have these immunisations. Taking steroids for long periods of time or in high doses can produce other damaging side-effects such as high blood pressure, diabetes, cataracts and muscle wasting. Now hundreds of patients who have experienced these and other side-effects as a result of taking steroids are claiming compensation for medical negligence.

In adults taking corticosteroids, the bones may be weakened, a condition known as osteoporosis, and in children, steroids can restrict growth. It is generally considered that giving steroids orally to children with eczema should be avoided because of these side-effects. Fortunately, there is an alternative steroid treatment which involves stimulating the child's own adrenal glands to increase their production of cortisol. This is achieved by giving injections of ACTH, which is short for Adrenalcorticotrophic hormone. This hormone is naturally produced in the pituitary gland at the base of the brain in response to stress or low blood levels of cortisol. It is then carried by the blood to the adrenal cortex, where it stimulates the production of cortisol. The benefit of this method of treatment is that ACTH does not suppress the function of the adrenal cortex, although it does share the other adverse side-effects of steroids, including the suppression of growth. This treatment may have another serious side-effect as well; the patient may have a potentially dangerous allergic reaction to this synthetic hormone. Most doctors prefer to administer steroids orally; however, ACTH is more appropriate in certain cases. If you suffer from severe atopic eczema or another inflammatory skin condition, it may be worth while looking into all other forms of treatment, including alternative therapies (see Chapter 4), before resorting to taking steroids. Again, it is important to emphasise the fact that all skin conditions, including eczema, are very individual and the same treatment will not suit everybody.

Wet Wrap Dressings

Wet wraps are rarely used in the UK but they are used frequently in other countries to treat children with extensive atopic eczema. Not only do they have a soothing effect on the eczema, they also make it difficult for the child to scratch the inflamed skin. Dr John Atherton, Consultant in Paediatric Dermatology at Great Ormond Street Hospital in London, recommends Tubifast® bandage for making the dressings, as it has a good degree of elasticity ensuring that it conforms well to the contours of the child's body without being too tight. It is also very absorbent and can maintain moisture for several hours. Tubifast® comes in five different widths depending on what area of the body you wish to bandage, and the strips should be cut to size before starting. First soak the strips of bandage in warm water; then apply them directly to the skin, having coated the skin with a rich moisturising cream or ointment, or a mild steroid cream. It is important to make sure that the child's skin is clean by bathing the child first. When applying the bandage, it is generally easier to start with the trunk before going on to cover each limb in turn.

If you have never put bandages on a child before, it is a good idea to experiment first by wrapping a favourite toy or teddy in bandages. There are a number of ways in which the ends of the bandages can be tidied away; perhaps the simplest way is to tie knots in the ends of the bandages. These dressings are best left on overnight and children should wear cotton clothing over them. Children are generally comfortable in these dressings and usually have no trouble sleeping.

PASTE BANDAGES

This type of bandage was originally made to treat leg ulcers in adults, but it can also be a useful method of treating atopic, varicose and discoid eczema, especially where the skin is thick and leathery. Those which are most effective contain coal-tar paste, but very raw areas of skin should be avoided as the high doses of coal tar can irritate and burn these tender places. If you find coal tar irritating, other paste bandages contain fossil-fish tar, ichthammol, which is much milder and is usually well tolerated by the skin. There are other paste bandages available on prescription containing soothing calamine lotion or the antibiotic clioquinol. When paste bandages are first applied, they have a refreshing, cooling effect and they can relieve much of the irritation as well as having various healing properties. The downside of using paste bandages is that they are messy, more so then wet wrap dressings.

A second type of bandage is needed to cover the wet paste bandages to keep them in place. You can use ordinary crêpe bandages for this purpose or, alternatively, there are special elasticated bandages (Coban®) which are non-adhesive, but are self-gripping. These allow air to pass through easily and they are available on prescription. Cotton gloves or mittens are useful for covering bandaged hands. These are also available on prescription or from the National Eczema Society (see Useful Addresses). Paste bandages can be left on the body for twenty-four hours and most children find them surprisingly comfortable.

Antibiotics

Antibiotics can be administered orally or topically to treat skin infections. The cracked, broken skin of eczema and other dry skin conditions is a perfect breeding ground for bacteria. The majority of skin infections are caused by the bacterium known as Staphylococcus aureus. Recent research carried out by Dr Michael Cork, Lecturer in Dermatology at the University of Sheffield, has revealed that this bacterium is present on all areas of eczematous skin, whether the skin is infected or not. For this reason, it may be more beneficial to treat eczema with a topical antibiotic/steroid combination instead of a topical steroid on its own although the use of such combinations is debatable. If your skin is infected, your doctor may take a swab (a small sample of your skin) before treating it with antibiotics. This will tell the doctor what type of bacterium is present and the swab can also be used to test the effects of different antibiotics.

The second most common bacterium responsible for causing skin infections is *Group A Staphylococcus*. This bacterium frequently causes sore throats so one of the signs that it is the cause of your skin infection is a sore throat or tonsillitis. Antibiotics are usually prescribed for a specific period such as five days or maybe even ten days and even if the infection clears before you have finished the tablets, you must continue to take them until the course is completed. This is to ensure that as many bacteria as possible are killed, otherwise the infection may return.

Antibiotics may also be administered topically to an infected area of skin. Topical antibiotics should be used for severe or extensive skin infections only when an antibiotic is given internally as well. Some antibiotics are too toxic to be given internally, but can be used safely on the skin. However, it is far better and easier to prevent an infection occurring in the first place than trying to combat it through a course of antibiotics. If you keep your skin clean and moisturise it regularly to maintain its natural protective barrier, the chances of it becoming infected are minimised.

Antihistamines

Histamine is a chemical substance which is released by the body into the skin during an inflammatory reaction. It is one of many substances, known as mediators of inflammation, which are released, but we know very little about the other mediators. It was previously thought that histamine was responsible for the itchy nature of inflammatory reactions such as eczema and so drugs which counter the effects of histamine, namely antihistamines, were often prescribed to eczema sufferers. The 'itch' of eczema can be very uncomfortable and distracting and sufferers often can't help scratching their skin and making their condition worse. However, it has become apparent over the years that the effects of antihistamines on eczema are more likely to be a result of the sedative effect they have, rather than any specific effect they have on the skin itself. This suggests that mediators other than histamine are responsible for the dreaded 'itch'. In support of this theory, it has been discovered that non-sedative histamines do not have the same beneficial effect as other antihistamines in reducing the 'itch'.

The fact remains, however, that oral antihistamines have had considerable success in stopping eczema sufferers aggravating their condition by scratching their skin. If you suffer badly from eczema, and are not put off by the drowsiness caused by taking antihistamines, then you may find a good deal of relief from taking them. Some may even find their sedative effect an added bonus, if sleeping is normally a problem, and there is no evidence that taking large doses of antihistamines over a long period of time is addictive. The best time to take antihistamines is at night at least an hour before going to bed, in order to avoid the 'hangover' effect the following morning. You should brush your teeth after taking an antihistamine syrup as these usually contain sugar. If you feel very sleepy, it is best not to drive. It is an intriguing fact that antihistamines can have the opposite effect on some children; stimulating them so that they are excitable during the day and sleepless at night. Other children may become drowsy, making them irritable and inattentive at school, so it is better to avoid antihistamines during the day.

There are a wide variety of sedative antihistamines available on prescription. High doses are often needed for the antihistamines to have any effect and many people find that continuous use reduces the beneficial effect of the drugs. To prevent this happening, take the antihistamines only when the eczema is particularly bad. If you take antihistamines every day, soon your body will become used to them and, when you need them most, you may find they no longer have the desired effect. Some antihistamines can make our skin sensitive to sunlight, so check with your doctor if the ones that you are taking have this effect. Eczema sufferers should not use antihistamine creams as they often cause allergic reactions.

Ultraviolet Therapy

Many dry skin, eczema and psoriasis sufferers find that their condition improves when exposed to sunlight or treatment with artificial sunlight. This should only be resorted to if your condition is very severe, as there is a worry that increased exposure to ultraviolet rays leads to the development of skin cancer. UVB rays on their own seem to have little effect as a treatment for atopic eczema, and natural sunlight – containing a mixture of UVA and UVB rays – is more beneficial. However, the most effective phototherapy treatment (PUVA) is known as psoralens photochemotherapy which involves a combination of UVA exposure and a drug, psoralens, which is given to the patient before exposure. Psoralens is a drug obtained from plants which dramatically magnifies the effect of UVA exposure. It can be given either by mouth, or sometimes it can be painted on to the skin as a lotion.

Oral PUVA has proved to be a very effective treatment of psoriasis and some cases of atopic eczema, especially in adolescents who have tried other treatments to no avail.

Unfortunately, it is an expensive and a difficult form of treatment to administer as the patient has to travel to regular treatment sessions as often as two or three times each week. However, the result is often very rewarding and the treatment has offered long-term improvement in eczema for many children. This treatment is not widely available because dermatologists are worried that it may lead to an increased risk in skin cancer and premature ageing of the skin and it may take as long as fifty years to establish whether the benefits of oral PUVA outweigh these possible risks.

The advantage of topical PUVA, over oral PUVA, is that it treats specific areas of skin as opposed to the whole body. Unfortunately, the topical applications of the drug can irritate the skin and the effect is less predictable. In any case, PUVA treatment is only given to patients with severe atopic eczema which covers almost the entire surface area of the skin, so oral PUVA is generally more appropriate. It is also possible to block out certain areas of the skin which do not need treatment when taking the drug orally, by covering these areas with clothing.

Cyclosporin

This is a fairly new drug treatment which is available for some people with atopic eczema. Like penicillin, it is produced by a fungus and was originally used in the 1970s to prevent the rejection of transplant organs. Dermatologists have used cyclosporin during the last five years to treat psoriasis and it has gained increased use recently as a treatment for other skin conditions, especially eczema. It works by suppressing strong allergic and immune reactions. Its most important activity in relation to eczema is the inhibition of production of cytokines by lymphocytes. Cytokines boost immunological and hence allergic reactions.

Cyclosporin is an extremely effective treatment for eczema although it will not work for all patients. Research has shown that nine out of ten people with eczema find that the itch and the appearance of the skin greatly improves when taking cyclosporin. Patients also benefit from an increase in the quality of their lives as they feel less embarrassed by their eczema and less distracted by soreness and itching. Those taking cyclosporin do not need any other treatment such as steroid creams, so there is no risk of side-effects from these treatments. The brand name for cyclosporin is Sandimmun which is usually taken in capsule form. It should not be used to treat mild forms of eczema because the side-effects would outweigh the benefits, and it is only used to treat adults.

No immune-suppressing drug should be taken lightly because of the serious side-effects. Those who suffer from cancer or have had cancer in the past are advised not to take this drug. Also anyone with a severe infection, such as tuberculosis, should not take cyclosporin because the immune system will not be strong enough to fight the infection. Extra consideration has to be paid to people with kidney disease, liver disease, high blood pressure, high blood cholesterol or diabetes. The side-effects of cyclosporin are, like those of steroids, dose related, so the higher the dose, the more likely you are to develop the side-effects. The side-effects are also more severe when taking the drug over a long period. The most important side-effect is a reduction in the efficiency of the kidneys whose role it is to cleanse the blood.

Cyclosporin can also increase blood pressure and raise the levels of sugar and cholesterol in the blood. The strangest side-effects which some patients experience are a swelling of the gums and 'pins and needles'. Some drugs can increase the side-effects of cyclosporin, so if you are taking cyclosporin and your doctor prescribes another drug, check that it is safe to have both treatments simultaneously.

Cyclosporin, like all other drugs, does not cure eczema and it is generally considered that the side-effects of taking a drug of this sort outweigh its benefits, except in special circumstances. Research is currently being carried out into the use of cyclosporin in cases of severe atopic eczema in order to establish what dose combines a good effect with a minimal amount of risk. We should know more about this drug in the next few years. At present, it is usually prescribed by dermatologists, not GPs, and never for children with eczema.

4

Complementary Therapies

Conventional treatments of eczema do not work for everyone and many patients taking them experience serious side-effects such as stunted growth and muscle damage. A study carried out by the National Eczema Society, involving more than three-thousand people with eczema, revealed that many eczema patients were dissatisfied with their initial consultations with both general practitioners and hospital doctors. Furthermore, only 44 percent of patients were satisfied with their conventional treatment (the majority were using topical steroids), and 16 percent of patients were dissatisfied. Those who have been unsuccessfully treated by conventional medicine are increasingly turning to complementary and alternative therapies which have gained a high profile in recent years.

One of the benefits of most alternative therapies is their holistic approach to illness. Chinese herbalists, homoeopaths and other holistic practitioners take into account the link between mind and body and this is particularly relevant to treating skin disorders, as they are often triggered by stress. Very few of the complementary therapies are accepted by the medical profession in Britain. However, many have had considerable success in treating a variety of conditions which do not respond well to conventional treatment.

Chinese Herbalism

Conventional doctors have been forced to acknowledge the Chinese herbalist's treatment of eczema because of the overwhelming success it has had in treating this exasperating and persistent condition. This is the only form of complementary therapy for eczema that is accepted by some conventional doctors. The Chinese have always used medicinal herbs to treat illness and Chinese herbalists often prescribe a mixture of herbs to treat eczema. The medical tradition of China is at least one thousand years older than any European medical traditions. China has a rich variety of medicinal plants and is probably the most expert country in the world in using them. Through centuries of use, the Chinese have gradually catalogued the different benefits and dangers of all these plants.

Chinese medicine works by restoring the balance between the various functions of the body. Each patient is given a different herbal remedy which is individual to his or her symptoms. The herbal remedy is usually prescribed in dry form and it is prepared by boiling the herbs in water for a specific time; the liquid is then strained, cooled and drunk. Chinese medicine seems antiquated to Western doctors, but the fact remains that it is successful in treating many conditions including eczema. In 1988 the National Eczema Society and several dermatologists became aware that some atopic patients who had not responded to conventional medicines had benefited from Chinese herbal remedies. These remedies had been prescribed by Dr Ding Hui Luo in Soho in London. Doctors trained in Western medicine then set out to study how effective and safe these Chinese medicinal herbs were in the treatment of atopic eczema. In order to do this, Dr Luo put together a standardised prescription of herbs to be tested, although she normally gives each patient an individual combination of herbs. This particular mixture was selected as suitable for patients with severe, widespread atopic eczema whose skin was very dry and not infected or exuding moisture.

The trials were carried out in London hospitals; one at Great Ormond Street and the other at the Royal Free in Hampstead. Tests were carried out during the trials to make sure that the patients' blood, kidneys and livers were healthy and remained so throughout the treatment. The dried herbs used in the trial were carefully chosen before being sealed in bags rather like tea-bags. Thirty-one adults and thirty-seven children completed the study and more than half of these people found that their eczema was better when they took the active herbal remedy than when they either took no herbal remedy or a dummy herbal remedy.

The trials lasted for eight weeks, during which time the patients experienced no harmful side-effects. The only side-effects suffered were reversible, such as headaches, nausea and stomach bloating. The two trials were then extended to a further twelve months to establish the long-term effects of taking the herbal remedy. The decoction continued to be effective and many patients were able to take it less often without this affecting their eczema. However, two children developed a change in their blood which suggested that the herbal remedy was having an adverse effect on their livers. When they were removed from the trial their blood returned to normal.

More studies are currently being carried out to establish how safe the herbal decoction is as a long-term treatment for eczema. Many people assume that because herbs are natural, they are automatically safe, but this is not always the case. However, many conventional treatments have harmful side-effects and bearing in mind the severe side-effects of taking oral steroids, herbal remedies seem to be a safer option for many people. No one knows exactly why this combination of herbs is so effective in treating eczema, although it is thought that it contains a number of active substances, including anti-inflammatory agents and immune-system suppressants. Research is now in progress to establish precisely what these active substances are.

The combination of herbs used in the trials is now available in granule form known as Zemaphyte. This is not a licensed product but some suitable eczema patients may be able to obtain the granules from their GP as a special prescription. However, some dermatologists believe that Zemaphyte should not be prescribed until further research has been carried out. For this reason, your dermatologist may not recommend this treatment for you. Zemaphyte should only be taken by those with severe, widespread atopic eczema whose skin is especially dry and not infected. Anyone taking this herbal remedy will need to do so for a number of months and should have blood and urine tests before and during their treatment. Be warned: it tastes horrible, but if it clears your eczema then this is well worth it. Research is being carried out at the time of writing to develop and test a new version of the treatment in pill form.

If you decide to approach a Chinese herbalist to treat your eczema then you must be warned that there are several unqualified people in Britain who offer Chinese herbal therapy. There have been a couple of deaths due to liver failure, said to have occurred after taking large doses of poisonous herbs. It is therefore important to consult a qualified and experienced herbalist. Unfortunately, there is no register of practitioners of Chinese medicine which would indicate those clinics run by properly trained people. The details of some known qualified Chinese herbalists are listed in the Useful Addresses at the back of this *Quick Guide*. Practitioners in traditional Chinese herbal medicine cannot prescribe Zemaphyte, but they may prescribe their own combination of Chinese medicinal herbs which will have to be paid for by the patient. Chinese herbal treatments should not be taken by those with liver or kidney disease or those taking any regular oral medication without discussion with a qualified and experienced practitioner.

Acupuncture

This is another traditional form of Chinese medical treatment and it has been used in China for about three thousand years. The Chinese believe that there is an invisible force, known as 'Qi', which flows between the limbs and the vital internal organs through channels called 'meridians'. They also believe that all illness reflects a disturbance in the natural harmony of the body, and acupuncture and other forms of Chinese medicine help to correct this. The nervous system is involved in the acupuncture process, with chemical substances being released in the brain and spinal cord. One of these substances is the adrenocorticotrophic hormone which helps to form a steroid. As we have seen, steroids have a beneficial effect on most skin diseases and acupuncture works by releasing the body's own steroids and helping the body to heal itself. Although acupuncture involves placing needles in strategic areas of the body, it is completely painless and, in children, alternatives can be used which involve the application of heat, pressure or laser beam.

There are no risks involved in acupuncture provided that the treatment is conducted by a qualified physician who is trained in the treatment of skin diseases by acupuncture. If you wish to have acupuncture you should see a qualified practitioner who has been trained and is well qualified (see Useful Addresses for details). A personal recommendation is best, but failing this, find a practitioner with many years' experience. Some doctors go on weekend courses in acupuncture, but obviously their level of expertise will not be the same as that of a specialist with lengthy experience.

Homoeopathy

This alternative approach to medicine developed in Europe during the nineteenth century. It is recognised by the medical profession in Britain as an accepted form of treatment for various conditions and it is established as a speciality within the NHS. There are two key ways in which homoeopathy differs from conventional Western treatment. First, homoeopaths have a holistic approach to their patients, taking into account the patient's lifestyle and state of mind as well as the physical symptoms. During an initial consultation, the homoeopath examines all aspects of an individual to draw up a clear picture of the person and his or her condition. Newcomers to homoeopathy often find the seemingly irrelevant questions on subjects other than their eczema rather bewildering. When treating eczema (as with all medical conditions) a homoeopath will separate the symptoms into three groups: local, mental and general. The local symptoms only apply to the disease, as to how itchy and inflamed the skin is, while the mental symptoms are stress and anxiety, etc.

Secondly, homoeopaths treat 'like with like'. This principal is based on the premiss that a substance which produces a set of symptoms in a healthy person can cure the same set of symptoms in a sick person. This can be interpreted in many ways; eczema, for example, is often treated with sulphur, a product of volcanoes, which are reminiscent of the hot, erupted skin of many eczema sufferers. Other treatments for eczema are arsenicum album which is a deadly poison in its undiluted form but safe in homoeopathic dilutions. Graphites (which are used to make pencils) are also sometimes used to treat eczema. In the case of urticaria (nettle rash), where the skin is swollen as if it were stung by a bee, the treatment is actual bee sting! Luckily the treatment is administered in small white sugar tablets. The idea of treating an illness with a substance which causes a similar condition itself seems strange, but it does work for many people.

Homoeopathic medicines do sometimes cause a reaction, making the condition worse before it gets better. This is known as an 'aggravation' and it is particularly common in skin complaints (15–20 percent). It is due to aggravations that homoeopaths reduce the size of their doses so that the remedies are given in minute quantities. This is achieved through a process known as 'potentisation' which dilutes the original substance ten times (1:10) or one hundred times (1:100). Homoeopathic medicines may be labelled 6c or 6th centesimal dilution. This means that the original substance, which is usually a herb, has been diluted 1:100, six times over. One of the main reasons why conventional doctors find it so hard to come to terms with homoeopathy, is the fact that the more diluted the original substance is, the more powerful it is. A high dilution of 30c is more potent than one of 3c, but it contains virtually no trace of the original substance. If a chemist were to analyse it, he or she would probably say that it consisted of water, alcohol (which is used to make the dilutions) and sugar (from the tablets) and nothing else!

Homoeopathic remedies work by stimulating the body's self-healing processes, and a lot depends on how long the patient has had eczema, how severe it is and what previous treatment he or she has had. Children often respond to homoeopathic treatment better than adults who have had eczema for a long time and who have used steroid creams. My own children have had several courses of homoeopathic treatment which have worked very well. However, you should not stop taking steroids or other treatments as soon as you start to take a homoeopathic treatment, but should reduce their use gradually with the advice of your doctor.

If you wish to find out more about where to get homoeopathic treatment, the details of the British Homoeopathic Association can be found at the back of this quick guide. It may be better to go to a homoeopathic doctor who has studied conventional medicine before specialising in homoeopathy. The qualification of non-medical practitioners is not properly regulated; however, those with the letters RSHom (Registered with the Society of Homoeopaths) after their names are trained. Some homoeopathic treatments are available on the NHS, although this service is limited, and there are five NHS homoeopathic hospitals in the U.K.

Evening Primrose Oil

There has been much interest in the humble evening primrose plant in recent years due to the constituents of the oil present in its seeds. Evening primrose oil has been used (with varying degrees of success) to treat a huge variety of medical conditions including premenstrual syndrome, diabetes, multiple sclerosis, rheumatoid arthritis, schizophrenia and eczema. The special ingredient of evening primrose oil is GLA, gamma-linolenic acid, which is a particularly important essential fatty acid. Essential fatty acids are found in vegetable, fish and nut oils. They are needed to form healthy cells and some are converted within us by enzymes into prostaglandins; hormone-like substances that regulate many functions within the body.

One of the most important essential fatty acids which is provided by our diet is linoleic acid. This is converted within the body into GLA but biochemists have discovered that in eczema sufferers, this conversion process is inactive and so GLA is not produced. We need GLA because it is a precursor to an important prostaglandin. Prostaglandins control cell-to-cell communication, strengthen the cell membranes and capillaries and boost the skin's impermeability, protecting it against moisture loss.

There have been numerous successful trials involving evening primrose oil as a safe treatment for eczema. Many eczema patients have experienced a noticeable improvement in the itchiness of their condition and it has also been demonstrated that taking evening primrose oil reduces the need for long-term treatment with steroids, antihistamines and antibiotics. Evening primrose oil is one of the few natural medicines which has been given a medical licence in this country and it is available on prescription in the form of Epogam capsules for adults and Epogam Paediatric twist-off-top capsules for children. Evening primrose oil is non-toxic and has no harmful side-effects, in contrast to the majority of other treatments for eczema. It is, therefore, suitable for young children, the elderly and breast-feeding women when many other treatments are not. However, it must be stressed that evening primrose oil does not work for everyone and it is not a fast-acting medicine; it may take as long as three months of daily use until it has any noticeable effect on the condition of the skin.

Echinacea

Echinacea is a purple flower which is widely grown in America and has been used there as a medicine for centuries. It is antibacterial and anti-inflammatory and is used by a number of natural therapists to treat a variety of skin disorders. Echinacea products have been used on the skin since the 1940s and extracts from the plant have been injected or given by mouth to those with dermatitis, eczema and psoriasis in order to improve the condition of their skin. There have been a number of clinical trials which have demonstrated the anti-inflammatory and wound-healing properties of echinacea. This wound-healing property of echinacea is thought to come from the polysaccharide content of the plant. Polysaccharides promote the production of new fibroblasts (cells which form connective tissue), and produce strong, healthy skin.

Other studies have revealed that echinacea can effectively treat numerous allergies, which may explain why it can dramatically improve the appearance of eczema and dermatitis in some people. Echinacea is available in tablet form, liquid extract or creams from chemists and health food centres. Echinacea extract is a good ingredient to look for when buying moisturisers for dry skin. One of the benefits of this natural remedy for inflammatory skin conditions is that it does not have the serious side-effects of steroids and other forms of traditional treatment. It is, in fact, an immune-boosting herb and helps to boost our body's immunity to infections and viruses. So not only should echinacea improve the condition of your skin, it should also help to protect you against the attack of flu and other viruses.

——— 5 ———

Food for Thought

Food Allergies

A healthy diet is essential for promoting cell renewal and producing strong skin. However, this is not as simple as it may seem, as it is not just a matter of eating lots of fresh fruit and vegetables and not so much of the dietary 'baddies' such as sugar, red meat or saturated fats. Some foods can irritate our digestive systems and others can cause allergies, and this can exacerbate eczema and other skin conditions. Allergies are caused by a faulty immune system. The body perceives some foods as enemies and it reacts in the same way as it does towards bacteria by producing antibodies to destroy them. Although the link between diet and skin disorders is discounted by some, leading dermatologists such as Professor Lowe agree that reactions can occur, with dairy protein and egg allergies being among the most common.

Food allergies are accompanied by a number of unpleasant symptoms which are often ignored, such as migraines, tiredness, depression, mood swings, constipation, stomach pains and hyperactivity. The same food can cause different allergies depending on where it comes into contact with the skin. Some foods may cause allergic reactions on the skin where contact is made, such as on the lips, but will have no effect internally; for example, you may have an allergic reaction to eating tomatoes whole, but tomato juice drunk through a straw may be fine. The form in which a food is eaten, ie raw or cooked, also makes a difference.

Sadly, it is often the case that the foods that we crave and enjoy the most are the ones we are allergic to. As an example, chocolate is one of the most common foods craved by psoriasis sufferers, although it often aggravates this skin condition. In the case of eczema sufferers and people with other skin disorders, a food allergy can prolong the condition for a considerable period of time. It is only in recent years that the public has become aware that we are what we eat and that many psychological and physical conditions can be improved or often cured through diet. Research has even shown that the severity of schizophrenia, a mental disease that affects many people in Britain, may be related to allergies. Tests carried out in France have linked violent behaviour of schizophrenics to coffee. Other tests carried out by probation officers in the north of England show that the behaviour of the offenders improved when their diet was changed from processed fast foods to balanced meals containing more fresh foods.

Food Intolerance

Food allergies are not the only aspect of our diets that we need to examine when treating eczema. Food intolerance is another important issue. The stomach, with the aid of the automatic (involuntary) nervous system, produces the continuous motion of the lining of the stomach. It moves slowly, so as to allow the food to mix with gastric juices as it is digested. The small pieces of semi-digested food are then mixed with bile and juice from the pancreas. The motions of the stomach lining carry the food through the small intestines to the colon before it eventually leaves the body. The skin and the nervous system are closely connected and this may explain why some foods which are difficult to digest may trigger eczema and other skin conditions. Food intolerance differs to food allergy in that it is dependent on how much of the food is consumed. People who are intolerant to cow's milk may find that drinking a little will have no effect, but those who are allergic to cows' milk generally react to even the smallest amounts.

Dairy products, often the cause of food allergies, are also difficult to digest. It is thought that the fat content of these foods tends to stick to the lining of the stomach, preventing us from making full use of the nutrients in the food. Many allergies and conditions such as eczema, psoriasis, migraine and arthritis can be triggered by dairy products. There are a number of foods which can provoke eczema such as wheat, nuts, tomatoes and fish, but dairy produce and eggs are the main culprits.

My son has inherited my own tendency to eczema and suffered quite badly as a baby. Fortunately, we discovered he was intolerant to milk and cheese, and his eczema cleared up when we removed these from his diet. However, I have been careful to supplement his diet with daily additional calcium supplies. This is especially important for young children who need a good, regular supply of calcium to build healthy teeth and bones. Anyone considering an exclusion diet of any type for their child should consult their doctor or a qualified nutritionist. For further information, read my *Quick Guide to Baby and Toddler Foods*, published by Boxtree.

It must be stressed that eczema may be provoked by other very different factors than diet alone. Some people may find that their eczema is mainly caused by dairy produce, in which case it is easy to improve the condition of their skin by simply avoiding milk and cheese, etc. For other eczema sufferers, the cause may be other unavoidable environmental factors such as house dust mites, in which case, cutting dairy produce from the diet will have no effect. Food allergies are very individual and for many eczema sufferers eating dairy produce, or other common allergy-causing foods, will not have any effect on the condition of the skin. However, statistics reveal that allergies to dairy produce, eggs and wheat are common in people with eczema, and if your eczema is particularly difficult to clear, then it is possible that your diet is exacerbating the condition.

Exclusion Diets

In order to establish if and what foods you are allergic or intolerant to, you need to take part in an exclusion diet, so called because it involves excluding certain foods from your diet in order to discover if this affects the condition of your skin. Keep a diary of the foods you eat, writing down any effects on the condition of your skin, either from eating the food or from excluding it from your diet. You may also like to make a note of any other common symptoms of allergy, such as headaches, stomach pains, depression, etc. It is important to remember that it can take several days before any effect of avoiding certain foods is observed. An intolerance to cows' milk is relatively common in atopic patients, so it may be best to start your exclusion diet by avoiding all cows' milk products for a week or two.

It is interesting to note that the Chinese, one of the largest populations in the world, do not include any dairy produce in their cuisine. Over the last hundred years or so in Britain, we have all been taught from an early age that milk is good for us, especially for children, as it is a rich source of calcium and protein. However, milk is high in saturated fat and there are other rich sources of calcium, such as nuts, seeds, pulses and many vegetables, such as broccoli. If you do cut dairy produce from your diet, it is important to ensure that you receive a good dose of protein and calcium either from other protein- and calcium-rich foods, or from a daily supplement. Other rich sources of protein are fish, meat, pulses and soya products.

Most of us have milk every day on our breakfast cereal, in our tea and coffee, in cheese sauces and in meals such as lasagne and moussaka. If you are allergic to cows' milk then you can substitute it with ewes' milk. This contains smaller molecules than cows' milk and is often easier to assimilate. It is possible to buy cheese, including Greek feta cheese, made from ewe's milk. Feta cheese can be used to make lasagne and other cheese dishes. Soya milk can also be used as a milk substitute in drinks. This is made from soya beans and it does not taste or smell like cows' milk, so children may not like it. Soya milk can also cause allergic reactions but this is not as common as those caused by cows' milk. Fortified soya milk formulas enriched with calcium can be bought for babies and young children who are allergic to cows' milk. Always choose unsweetened varieties as even lightly sugared blends can rot young teeth.

Hydrolysate formulas can also be bought from chemists. These contain a 'predigested' form of the main proteins in cows' milk. The whole proteins are broken down into peptides which destroy any antigenic elements, so that the formula is extremely unlikely to cause allergic reactions. Hydrolysate formulas contain all the other components of cows' milk such as fats, carbohydrates, vitamins and minerals.

Another alternative to cows' milk is goats' milk. However, goats' milk is not subject to the strict hygiene controls that cows' milk is exposed to in order to guard against harmful bacteria (although some health-food enthusiasts advocate that this is a good thing). Goats are usually hand-milked instead of machine-milked and this increases the probability of contamination. Goats' milk is rarely pasteurised with heat treatment, while cows' milk is nearly always pasteurised. For these reasons it is best to try soya and hydrolysate milk as a substitute for cows' milk first. If you do not like these milk formulas and decide to try goats' milk, it is available in dried, refrigerated or frozen form from health food shops and some supermarkets. Dried or refrigerated goats' milk is best. It is important to check on the packaging to see if the milk has been pasteurised; if it has not, boil it for two minutes, allow to cool, and then drink. The milk will taste worse after boiling and some of the nutrients, particularly folic acid, will be reduced. Goats' milk should not be given to babies under six months of age.

Eggs are also often the source of food allergies and some eczema sufferers experience an immediate reaction to them. Unlike milk, they can be eliminated from the diet without causing any harm or potential malnutrition. They can easily be replaced with other protein foods such as fish, pulses, or meat. If you want to cut out egg from your diet, avoid 'egg substitutes' which contain the egg protein ovalbumin. You must also avoid dried egg powder, egg yolk, egg white, egg albumin and egg lecithin. Vegetarians and vegans will have to make sure that they are getting enough protein through pulses and algae. A dietitian may also recommend that chicken should be included in the exclusion list as chicken contains some of the amino acid which are also present in egg protein.

Wheat can also provoke eczema and other skin conditions and it is, unfortunately, one of the most difficult types of food to eliminate from the Western diet. We have wheat in almost every meal, from toast and cereal at breakfast and sandwiches at lunchtime, to pasta dishes in the evening. Many people are allergic to wheat without ever realising it and the symptoms can range from weight-gain to depression. If your eczema never seems to improve or if you have other symptoms such as fatigue and depression, then a wheat intolerance may be to blame. Those with persistent chronic eczema are sometimes advised to change to a wheat-free diet. Wheat is an important carbohydrate, which is the main source of energy in our diet, so it is important that we eat other carbohydrates such as rice. Fortunately, there are many wheat substitutes including buckwheat, millet, potato flour, rye, rice and soya flour. Tasty bread made from rye is available from large supermarkets and health food shops.

Let me re-emphasise that before embarking on an exclusion diet either for yourself or your child, make sure that you seek the advice of a qualified dietitian as you will suddenly be cutting a rich source of vital nutrients out of your diet. If you are eliminating dairy produce, which is a good source of protein and calcium, you must make sure that you are getting enough protein from other sources such as pulses, fish or meat, and enough calcium from nuts, pulses and vegetables. Growing children need more calcium than the rest of us to form strong, healthy bones and it might be advisable to give your child a calcium supplement if he or she is allergic to dairy produce.

Other Irritating Foods

Naturopath Jan de Vries has treated several thousand patients with various skin diseases and he recommends that eczema sufferers with food allergies should also avoid all pig products, ie pork sausages, bacon or ham, as well as refined white sugar and flour, spices, alcohol and chocolate. He also recommends that those with food allergies eat liberal amounts of fruit and vegetables and drink plenty of mineral water. Processed food containing colourings, such as tartrazine, and preservatives, such as benzoate, should also be avoided as these can cause irritation and may aggravate eczema. Jan de Vries also believes that most eczema sufferers are deficient in essential fatty acids. This is not hard to believe, as our modern diet seems to consist mostly of processed food which is depleted of many of the nutrients essential for good health and strong skin. Dermatologist Dr Roland Payne also warns against icy or hot food and drink, and against specific foods including lemons, limes, grapefruit, salt, peppers, raw onions, horseradish, pickles, vinegar, mustard and any other salty or spicy food.

—6—

Lifestyle and Environmental Factors

The environment in which we live and the substances which we come into contact with every day affect our health and the condition of our skin. On a very basic level, living in grimy cities clogs the pores of our skin with dirt and this upsets its gentle chemistry. This is the least of the worries felt by eczema and dermatitis sufferers. These skin disorders are aggravated by many factors including everyday objects, such as plants and synthetic clothing, which most of us perceive as harmless. This is particularly true of dermatitis, a dry skin condition which manifests itself in inflammatory reactions to certain substances.

Dermatitis

ALLERGIC CONTACT DERMATITIS

Our skin can be allergic to substances that are hard to avoid in daily life, for example washing clothes in a certain liquid detergent or washing powder may cause your skin to react when it comes into contact with the clean clothes. Other causes of allergic contact dermatitis are common plants such as chrysanthemums and primulas. Cosmetics can also cause allergic reactions. The symptoms of allergic contact dermatitis usually appear between two to three days after the skin has come into contact with the irritating substance, although it can take as long as two weeks for the allergen to penetrate through to the dermis. This often makes it difficult to pin-point the exact cause of the allergic reaction. Below are some of the substances which can cause allergic reactions in the skin:

Allergen	Possible source
nickel	ear-rings, watch straps, bra fastenings, zips and jewellery, coins, kitchen tools, pots and pans
aluminium	deodorants
cobalt	cement, inks
chromates	cement, anti-corrosives, all leather, printing
dyes	hair colourants and clothing, particularly those containing paraphenylenediamine (PPD)
rubber	elastic, shoes and gloves
epoxy resin	glues
antiseptics	chloroxyenol (Dettol), chlorhexidine (Savlon)
preservatives	creams and lotions (pharmaceuticals, cosmetics and toiletries)

IRRITANT CONTACT DERMATITIS

Irritant contact dermatitis is triggered by a wide variety of substances, often with no predictable time interval between contact and the resulting rash. Its severity varies with the quantity, concentration, and length of exposure to the irritating substance. In cases of irritant contact dermatitis, the rash will only appear in the area of skin exposed to the substance, unlike allergic dermatitis where the rash can appear in areas of the body that may not have been touched by the allergen. In acute conditions of irritant dermatitis, the skin will become red and blister, causing great discomfort. The damage occurs gradually where the skin is exposed to a mild irritant over a long period of time. First, the keratin layer of skin becomes damaged which allows the skin to dehydrate, and as more water evaporates through the skin, the more damaged the keratin layer becomes. Dermatitis can also be itchy.

PREVENTION AND TREATMENT

The best method of treating contact dermatitis is to identify the substance which causes the allergy or the irritation in order to avoid contact with it in the future. The offending substances tend to fall into the following six categories:

* clothing
* cosmetics
* household objects such as cleaning detergents
* occupational objects such as petroleum products
* plants
* medicines

Clothing

The most common substances which cause dermatitis are organic dyes, rubber in elastic, and nickel in buttons, zips and hooks. Nylon tights and stockings may also cause a rash on the inner surface of the upper part of the thighs, backs of the knees and on the feet and toes, although this is generally thought to be due to the dye rather than the nylon. Nappy rash is another form of dermatitis caused by the prolonged wearing of wet nappies, usually due to the ammonia in the urine rather than the nappy itself.

Cosmetics

Certain chemicals in cosmetics may cause irritant or sensitising reactions. Some of the most sensitising chemicals are para-phenylenediamine (PPD), which is a hair dye, and formalde-hyde which is used in nail varnishes, perfumes, eye make-up and in some of the preservatives and fragrances used in skincare creams. Dermatitis caused by cosmetic products affects the skin around the eyelids, neck and ears. It is interesting to note that the skin may become sensitised in areas other than where the product is applied. For example, in the case of nail varnish, the eyelids, neck and face may show a reaction, while the skin around the nails is fine.

Household objects

It is not surprising that the hands are far more afflicted by contact dermatitis than the rest of the body and we should really take more care of them than we generally do. We would never consider treat-ing the skin on our faces in the same way that we treat our hands. If you do a lot of housework or cleaning at work, then you will be putting your hands through hell on a daily basis unless you wear protective rubber gloves. Detergents are the most common cause of contact dermatitis in the form of soaps and harsher cleaning agents. The very action of cleaning something with detergents literally rubs the harsh chemical ingredients into the skin, so that they penetrate through the stratum corneum to the new skin beneath. However, wearing rubber gloves is not always the answer to this problem as they can also cause dermatitis.

Occupational objects

Many professionals are exposed to harsh chemicals daily at work which can cause contact dermatitis. Mechanics, hairdressers, engineers, nurses, domestic workers and housewives are all at risk from exposure to petroleum products, detergents, oils, solvents, paint constituents or cement. These irritant substances damage the protective keratin layer and penetrate deep into the skin causing an inflammatory reaction. Many people who develop dermatitis are atopics, who may have had eczema in childhood. If this is the case, then avoid exposing your body to irritants. Do not fret, however, if your job involves working with chemicals which irritate your skin, as using emollient barrier creams can help prevent the onset of dermatitis.

Plants

Perhaps surprisingly, some ordinary garden plants can be a cause for concern. The most common plants responsible for causing dermatitis are ivy, primula, chrysanthemums, celery, tulips, daffodils, narcissi and clematis. Gardeners should take care with these plants and wear gardening gloves.

Medicines

There are many types of skin rash caused by drugs; one common reaction is photosensitivity caused by medicines taken internally, and another is a photoallergic reaction caused when certain drugs are applied to the skin, causing reactions at the point of application (these include antihistamines, some chemical sun creams, coal tar and its derivatives and local anaesthetics).

HOW TO ESTABLISH THE CAUSE OF DERMATITIS

One of the clues to the cause of dermatitis is the location of the rash on the body. The head, neck and face area tend to be affected by cosmetics and may be indirectly affected by nickel. Plants such as primula (the common primrose) can cause a reaction to appear on the face. Discovering the cause of dermatitis on the hands is not so straightforward as our hands touch practically everything and so the number of substances which could be the irritant or allergen is enormous. Detergents and other cleaning agents, petrol, oil and cement are the most common causes of irritation. The arms are often affected by house dust mites and plants, while the armpits may be affected by deodorants and other cosmetics and clothing. The torso is usually sensitised through contact with metal clips, elasticated underwear and medication. Finally, the feet may develop dermatitis as a result of wearing certain shoes, socks or tights.

Eczema

Allergy is another main trigger of eczema in atopic patients. One of the main causes of allergic reactions in eczema sufferers is house dust mites. These microscopic creatures are related to ticks and spiders and, as they are only about a third of a millimetre long, they are not visible to the naked eye. No matter how much effort you put into cleaning your home and dusting, every house contains millions of these tiny creatures. And, although they may be small, the dust mite is the single most important cause of allergy in Britain. Dust mites love the damp which is why they are so abundant in our wet climate. These little critters feed on dead skin flakes and eczema sufferers find themselves in a *Catch 22* situation as they shed more than the rest of us. It is thought that the dust mite droppings contain a protein which is the main cause of the allergy. House dust mites live for about six weeks and during this time a female mite can produce up to eight eggs. It takes three to four weeks for the eggs to develop into adult mites, so it is easy to see why they are so difficult to eradicate. Each adult mite can produce up to forty droppings every day and so it is impossible for eczema sufferers to avoid these.

Fortunately, however, there are a few precautions we can take to limit the number of dust mites we are exposed to.

PRECAUTIONS

* House dust mites thrive in warm, moist environments and they live in soft furnishings such as mattresses, carpets and sofas. Old mattresses should be covered with an air-tight plastic liner to keep the mites and their droppings at bay. If you need to buy a new mattress, Slumberland produce a range with a special interliner that protects against house dust mites and their droppings. Solid foam mattresses are better than those which are interior sprung and water beds are the least likely to harbour house mites. Avoid having padded headboards on your bed as these are difficult to keep dust-free. Children with eczema should not sleep in the bottom bunk of a bunk bed as dust mite droppings from the mattress above may fall on to the sleeper below.

* Bedding made from man-made fibres is least likely to attract house dust mites, although, unfortunately, many eczema sufferers find that these synthetic fibres can irritate their skin condition. If you have the time and the energy, sheets and pillowcases should be washed daily and duvets should be washed once a week. You can also buy anti-allergy pillows and duvets which can be washed in very hot temperatures. All bedding, including mattresses, should be aired regularly. Mattresses should be vacuumed regularly, at least once a week.

* House dust mites also love soft toys. So if your child has eczema, try to limit the amount of soft toys, wash them

regularly and try not to let your child take the toys to bed. For cases of severe childhood eczema, soft toys can be stored in the freezer and thawed before bedtime, as house dust mites perish in sub-zero temperatures.

* Carpets gather huge amounts of dust and rugs are the same and so should be avoided. If you do have rugs, make sure that they are small and washable. Wooden floors and lino tiles are the easiest types of flooring to keep dust-free. Professor Nicholas Lowe advises his patients to remove carpets altogether from bedrooms.

* If you really want to avoid house dust, then keep your furnishings plain and simple with few ornaments, as this will make dusting easier. Textured wallpaper, plants and books are all great dust-gatherers.

* Keep clothing and toys in a cupboard or other dust-free environment when you are not using them.

* Dust all surfaces at least once a week with a damp duster, as dry dusting releases mite droppings into the atmosphere.

* If you have eczema, wear PVC gloves over cotton inner gloves for any cleaning.

* You can buy vacuum cleaners which are designed specifically for those with dust allergies. There is a medical vacuum cleaner called Medivac, which claims to have an absolute dust filtration system and conforms to British Standards. Electrolux also produce a vacuum cleaner with an advanced air-filtration system, Electrolux Airstream 1000. Vorwerk is another advanced German-made model. Registered eczema and asthma patients can re-claim the VAT on these appliances to help reduce their cost. Conventional vacuum cleaners only retain the large dust particles and the sub-microscopic particles leak through the filter system and settle again on furniture. It is best to wear a

mask while hoovering as every time you switch on the cleaner, dust particles are released into the atmosphere. Change the hoover bags frequently.

* Keeping the air as dry as possible discourages dust mites and moulds from breeding, and installing extractor fans in the bathroom and kitchen is a good idea. Dehumidifiers can also help, but the down-side of living in a dry environment is that your skin is more likely to become dry and this can also exacerbate eczema. It is a matter of weighing up the pros and cons of living in a dry atmosphere; if the condition of your skin improves in a drier atmosphere, then you should keep it dry. You can always apply a moisturising cream two or three times a day to counteract your environment.

* Electronic ionisers and air cleaners may also help to keep the dreaded dust mites at bay. In the natural outdoor environment the electrostatic balance of positive and negative ions in the air is approximately equal. The situation indoors is somewhat different; the negative ions are depleted by air pollution dust, tobacco, heating, televisions and computers. This positively charged air attracts and holds suspended dust particles which can aggravate eczema and dry skin. An ioniser releases negative ions into the room which restore the neutral electrical balance. Air cleaners filter the air and reduce the levels of tobacco smoke, dust and pollen in the atmosphere. For details on where to buy these and other dust-reducing products see the Useful Addresses section of this *Quick Guide*.

CLOTHING

Man-made fibres such as nylon and polyesters, as well as wool, often irritate the skin, and if you have eczema, these fibres can make your skin incredibly itchy. Cotton is the best material to wear, whether you have a skin disorder or just dry skin. It can be difficult to find clothes made from 100 percent cotton, as the majority of clothes are made from mixed fibres. However, some of these materials may not irritate the skin if they have a high cotton content. Tight clothes should not be worn as these can make the skin hot and itchy. When choosing clothes, make sure the material is smooth and soft and watch out for rough seams, elastic, labels, zips, etc which could irritate the skin. In winter, wear cotton clothes next to the skin and then put on warmer material over these undergarments. Remember that jumpers and clothes worn over the cotton may touch the wrist area and eczema may develop here as a result. Clothes are often dyed or coated in a special finish and this can cause allergic contact eczema. To avoid this, always wash your new clothes before wearing them in order to get rid of the finish and any excess dye. You can obtain a list of stockists of cotton goods as well as suppliers of house dust mite prevention bedding from the National Eczema Society. Cotton-On is one example of an excellent cotton clothing mail-order supplier, specialising in soft cotton clothing (including underwear and nightclothes) for all ages (see Useful Addresses).

FUNGI AND MOULDS

The spores from fungi and moulds can also be the cause of allergic reactions. Mould grows outside on plants, trees, and on compost and other damp areas, but it also grows inside in damp rooms. Fungi and moulds love damp conditions, especially areas which are dark, humid, poorly ventilated and which have heavy condensation. If you have a large damp patch on your wall and you leave some clothes or shoes next to it, they will soon become mouldy. A friend of mine once had fungi growing on the floor in her car because it was so damp and rusty. The best way to avoid contact with mould and fungi is to stay away from damp areas. Keep your house well ventilated to keep moulds, fungi and dust mites at bay. This can, of course, be difficult if the weather outside is very cold or if opening windows means that you will breathe in too much pollen or other allergens. It is a matter of choosing the lesser evil. 'High efficiency' particle air filter systems can effectively reduce any build-up of pollen and mould spores, particularly in bedrooms.

Moulds and fungi also grow on some foods such as beans, grains, dried fruit and apples so make sure to check these products are clean before you eat them. Those who are sensitive to moulds and fungi should avoid eating mushrooms (a fungus) and 'mouldy' cheese such as stilton, brie and camembert.

POLLEN

For eczema, hay fever and asthma sufferers, high pollen counts can make summer a miserable time of the year. There are two types of pollen which can exacerbate eczema: tree and grass pollen. If your eczema gets worse from the beginning of April until the end of May, then tree pollen is to blame, but if your condition is worse from the beginning of May until the end of July, then you are probably allergic to grass pollen. You may, of course, be unfortunate enough to be allergic to both types of pollen. Sadly, the most effective way of avoiding pollen is by remaining inside and shutting all windows. When outside, you should avoid grassed areas and if you do come into contact with pollen by mistake, you should shower immediately, rub an emollient into your skin, and then put on fresh clothes.

One of the newest forms of treatment, Nasaleze, is a unique grade of vegetable cellulose powder which, when applied to the nostrils, is converted into a gel, forming a protective barrier over the nasal mucosa. This gel-like barrier traps and inactivates any allergens – such as pollen and house dust mites – which enter the nose and so helps to prevent any allergic reactions. It is said to be effective for up to twelve hours, after which it disperses naturally.

PETS

Most furry pets are likely to trigger eczema because their hair, saliva and urine contain antigenic proteins. Shed skin (dander) is the main source of antigen, and cats and dogs shed large amounts of skin in the home. The dander is broken up and small particles become airborne and are spread quickly throughout the home in the same ways as dust. Human and animal skin is food for dust mites. It is best to allow pets only in certain rooms of the house which can easily be cleaned, and never allow them in the bedroom. An allergy to animals may not be immediately noticeable and it can be some time after a person has come into contact with an animal, that the reaction develops. The less fur a pet has, the less likely it is to cause a problem. For example, smooth-coated Burmese cats cause less of a reaction than longer-haired chinchillas. All pets should be shampooed regularly and longer-haired dogs should be gently vacuumed using a brush attachment (most dogs actually like it!). If you have eczema and are thinking of getting a pet, it is worth while seeing how you react to other people's pets first.

TOBACCO SMOKE

The National Eczema Society suggest that cigarette smoke should be banned from a house where an eczema sufferer lives. Tobacco smoke contains a number of toxic substances which irritate the eyes, nose and lungs, and exposure to the smoke increases the probability of new allergies developing, and of asthma being triggered in those with eczema.

Glossary

Allergen – a substance which causes an allergic reaction.

Antibodies – a special kind of blood protein that the body releases in response to the presence of antigens in order to render their attack harmless.

Antigen – a substance that the body regards as potentially dangerous.

Atopy – a tendency to become allergic to common and usually harmless environmental substances and to develop conditions such as eczema, asthma and hay fever.

Capillaries – thin, narrow blood vessels which enable oxygen, water, salts and other substances to pass between the blood and body tissue.

Diuretic – something that increases the volume of urine produced by promoting the excretion of salts and water from the kidneys.

Essential fatty acids – polyunsaturated fatty acids which are termed 'essential' as they are required for good health. They must be supplied by the diet as they cannot be synthesised by the body.

Fibroblasts – cells which form connective tissue and which produce collagen, elastic fibres and reticular fibres.

Lesions – tissue which has been damaged by disease or wounding.

Photosensitivity – an abnormal reaction by the skin to sunlight.

Sensitisation – when the body develops an allergy, an individual becomes sensitised to a particular allergen and reaches a state of hypersensitivity and tends to respond abnormally to foreign substances, whether they are harmful or not.

Topical – local, meaning that the drug is applied directly to the area of the skin which needs treating.

Wheals – temporarily red or pale raised areas of the skin that often itch severely and which sometimes indicate an allergy.

Useful Addresses

100 Per Cent Cotton
22 Hambledon Court
Holmwood Gardens
Wallington
Surrey SM6 0HN
Tel: 0181 669 6028
Made-to-measure clothing

The Alternative Centre for Psoriasis and Eczema Sufferers
The White House
Roxby Place
Fulham
London SW6 1RS
Tel: 0171 381 2298

Beauty Care and Camouflage Service
The British Red Cross Service
Grosvenor Crescent
London
SW1 7EI
Tel: 0171 235 5454

The British Homoeopathic Association
27A Devonshire Street
London W1N 1RJ
Tel: 0171 935 2163

British Medical Acupuncture Society
68–69 Chancery Lane
London WC2 1AF
Tel: 01925 730727

Cosmetic, Toiletry and Perfumery Association
35 Dover Street
London
W1X 3RA
Tel: 0171 491 8891

Cotton-On Ltd
Monmouth Place
Bath
Avon BA1 2NP
Tel: 01225 461155
Cotton clothing

The Healthy House
Cold Harbour
Ruscombe
Stroud
Gloucestershire GL6 6DA
Tel: 01453 752216
Mail-order anti-allergy catalogue

The Homoeopathic Trust
2 Powis Place
London WC1N 3HT
Tel: 0171 837 9469

Medivac Healthcare Products
Bollin House
Riverside Works
Manchester Road
Wilmslow
Cheshire SK9 1BJ
Tel: 01625 539401
Vacuum cleaners and bedding products

The National Eczema Society
163 Eversholt Street
London NW1 1BU
Tel: 0171 388 4097

The National Institute of Medical Herbalists
41 Hatherley Street
Winchester
Hampshire SO22 6RR
Tel: 01962 68776

Slumberland Plc Medicare Division
Salmon Fields
Oldham
Greater Manchester OL2 6SB
Tel: 0161 628 5293
Health Seal range of bedding products

Index